FOODS
—FOR—
THOUGHT

Understanding the Impact of Diet
and Lifestyle on Mental Health

FOODS FOR THOUGHT
Understanding the Impact of Diet and Lifestyle on Mental Health

Paperback (ISBN): 978-1-7363717-0-1
Ebook (ISBN): 978-1-7363717-1-8

Editor: *Serena Howlett*
Indexer: *Jason Pawloski and Almira Joy Bautista*
Interior/layout designer: *Almira Joy Bautista*
Cover Designer: *Charala*

FOODS

—FOR—

THOUGHT

Understanding the Impact of Diet and Lifestyle on Mental Health

JASON PAWLOSKI, MS, RDN

CONTENTS

ACKNOWLEDGEMENTS

Being my first attempt at writing a book, this journey demanded more time and energy than I had anticipated and bargained for. I'm forever grateful to those who showed support during this busy two years of writing and bringing this idea to fruition and all the way to publication. Much love and thanks for my mother, Pati, and my nephew, James, who have encouraged and inspired me on this journey.

I also would not have been able to make this book happen without some talented and passionate help of others. Thank you, Serena Howlett, for your expertise and guidance editing my first book, you've added value and clarity to my vision and it was a joy to work with you. Much thanks to Almira Joy Bautista for your patience and skills with book interior layout design. Thank you, Charala, for your design mastery and for going above and beyond to execute my vision of a great front cover.

Part of my inspiration to write this book also came from the amazing, integrated team of healthcare professionals that I've had the chance to work with over past few years. Though I can't mention all of them here, thank you kindly to Ed Pinnow, Dr. Anupama Trighatia, Tonjua Sibley, and Tracie Johnson-Wagner. Each of you supported me and provided resources along my journey turning an idea into a book. I sincerely appreciate you and your dedication to a challenging population that we serve in Arizona.

FOREWORD

I met Jason several years ago when he came to my behavioral health residential facility to provide a class on nutrition. I distinctly remember feeling somewhat sorry for him because I knew the patients he was about to address. Some were hard-core addicts with co-occurring mental health issues that were just days clean from opiates and myriad other substances. I knew the last thing they would be interested in hearing is someone talking to them about their diets and nutrition. Wow, was I wrong!

Not only did Jason grab their attention, but after listening to him the patients wanted to work with clinicians to add nutritional issues to their behavioral health treatment plans. I was so shocked at the patients' positive response I decided to sit in the next time Jason did a class. I soon discovered that Jason has a gift to make nutritional concepts very easy to understand.

Since then, Jason has helped me achieve my nutritional goals for overall health as well as for participation in endurance sports. Through his support I have achieved a balance of mind and body that I never knew was possible.

When I found out that Jason was writing a book I was definitely excited. This book does not disappoint! The information is presented in a responsible manner, scientifically backed yet written in a way that is clear and easy to understand. I hope you find it as interesting, affirming and motivating as I have.

Edward Pinnow, LISAC, Program Director, residential treatment facility, Phoenix, AZ

PREFACE

Food and nutrition — and making healthy lifestyle choices — haven't always come easy to me. It wasn't until junior college with an undecided major that I became interested in fitness and then became certified as a personal trainer. During this time studying general education while working as a trainer, I became inspired to learn about nutrition and lifestyle changes, and to become qualified to share knowledge with the ultimate intention of empowering others to take charge of their health outcomes. Considering that I was never a "good student" academically throughout elementary or high school years, once I reached college I realized that I had to work much harder than ever before in order to accomplish what I sought. I wanted to become a registered dietitian and use my knowledge to improve the lives of people living with chronic illness and depression, help people overcome unhealthy eating habits and guide people to healthier, happier lives.

For the past five years I have been a registered dietitian nutritionist practicing in Arizona. After my first two years of clinical practice in Yuma, a few years ago, I returned to my hometown of Phoenix to focus my clinical work on helping those with mental health disorders and/or substance abuse disorders, along with chronic illnesses. I have a B.S. in Dietetics and M.S. in Human Nutrition. In my work as a clinician, I collaborate with an integrated health care team to provide optimal care for patients who have mental health diagnoses and serious mental illnesses. As a guest speaker, I lead group therapy discussions on the role of nutrition for mental health and substance abuse recovery. I also have eight years of experience as a certified personal trainer.

After years of helping thousands of people work towards their health goals, one thing has become clear to me. Everyone — regardless of their unique limitations, challenges, and barriers — has the ability to take charge of their personal health, learn to be responsible for their daily choices and understand how these daily choices directly and indirectly impact not just physical well-being, but also mental well-being.

This book is not meant to be the solution to your complex gut health and mental health problems. Rather it's meant to explain that lasting relief, for many, can be found when you commit to lifestyle changes, and, for some, follow a strict gut healing protocol designed by a physician and/or registered dietitian nutritionist who has specialized training in integrative and functional medicine.

INTRODUCTION

Before talking about food, let's take a moment to recognize that improving overall health — and in particular mental health — is not always as simple as eating healthy and exercising regularly. This book is not meant to be a simple answer or a fix to existing mental health problems, or a one-size-fits-all approach to treat anxiety or depression. Rather, this book is about helping you understand the significance of how your everyday choices and activities may be a major contributor to an underlying abnormality in your mood. This includes your choices about what you eat and drink, or perhaps more importantly what you do not eat and drink (enough of). It's also about helping you understand the role that other lifestyle factors play in your mental health, whether with regard to developing diseases or better managing existing mental illness. Identifying how these lifestyle factors contribute to illness is just the first step to finding lasting solutions to improve your quality of life.

This book is about presenting potential solutions to digestive problems (for some, not for all), weight loss or maintenance, and perhaps even better for some people, to feel significant improvements in mood, depression, and anxiety. Furthermore, it's about exploring and understanding lasting, life-changing individualized approaches toward improving your overall physical and mental health. Contrary to beliefs commonly held in the past that mental health is separate or distinct from the health of the rest of the body, we now know that we cannot separate physical and mental health.

Considered the final frontier of scientific discoveries by some experts, the brain is a complex organ that neuroscientists still have much to learn about— as they continue to acquire knowledge in the field of neuroscience in general. Likewise, the intestines are part of a complex organ system that experts in the broader field of gut health still have much to learn about. But one thing that has become clearer over the past couple of decades is the critical link between the health of the brain and the intestines in relation to diet and lifestyle.

In the busy, fast-paced, and oftentimes stress-inducing society that most of the developed world lives in today, there are several different aspects of overall wellness that one should be mindful of to promote optimal health — including mental health — and thrive as humans are meant to. This is why I couldn't simply cover the main topic of a healthy diet for optimal mental well-being, and must also explore other lifestyle factors. I will explore each of these key concepts for wellness and self-care in a special section at the end of the book. Sure, considering all of this might seem overwhelming to some. However, your health improvement journey is unique. There may be some of these concepts of wellness and self-care that you already do well, while other concepts you recognize you need to work on.

There's no doubt that your daily food and nutrition intake impacts mood and mental health. The term "standard American diet" (SAD) is used to describe the typical nutrient-deficient diet consumed by so many Americans. A nutritionally inadequate diet can lead to and can even worsen mental illness; however, a balanced and nutrient-dense diet can help prevent and even treat it. In those with mental illness, a diet deficient in critical nutrients and/or loaded with highly processed foods and refined carbohydrates and low in fibrous plant-based whole foods that provide essential nutrients is common.[1] For a person existing on this nutrient-deficient diet, who suffers from clinical depression and digestive problems, such as irritable bowel syndrome, improvement in diet may play a significant role in improving mood. The link between digestive health and mental health is becoming increasingly strong and so we cannot separate the two. In other words, what impacts your digestive health is likely to impact your mental health over time.

Mental illnesses are complex matters that for most people cannot be simply explained by inadequate food and nutrient intake. Besides diet and genetics, some other factors that likely contribute to the increasing incidence of mood disorders, such as major depression and bipolar disorder, include a sedentary lifestyle, lack of adequate social support, inadequate sunlight exposure, and an overall lack of connection with nature.[2] This book will explore the food-mood link in detail to help you understand how and why a nutritious diet is essential for mental well-being. Although your dietary intake may not be the cause or cure to a mental health disorder, it may be a big piece of the puzzle in improving symptoms and achieving the best health you can.

I am going to discuss several different pieces of the puzzle you can use to help improve your overall health and quality of life. With a recently advanced understanding of the link between the health of the brain and the health of the intestinal tract, not only can we enhance conventional modes of treatment and improve outcomes for mental illness, but we can also better facilitate weight loss in those who have struggled with continued weight gain or an inability to lose weight after multiple past attempts.[3]

In Part I, I will talk about depression and other mental health disorders that may be influenced by diet, the effects different dietary patterns can have on mood, mental health, and inflammation. In Part II, you will learn about the "gut-brain axis", certain gastrointestinal disorders that often pose obstacles to weight loss, how to maintain gut health, and the pros and cons of intermittent fasting, ketogenic diets, and supplements. In Part III, you will learn to craft your best plan for improved digestion and mental health (your *Foods for Thought Game Plan*). Finally, I will offer you real-life solutions to take charge of your health, lose weight (or maintain a healthy weight), and adopt nutritional and lifestyle changes — ultimately, to help you live a healthier, longer and more fulfilling life.

HEALTH OF A NATION: HOW DID WE GET HERE?

Relatively recently humans underwent dramatic lifestyle changes in a short period of time: not only have the food staples we subsist on changed, but our social support systems and level of physical activity (or lack thereof) have also changed to accommodate modern lifestyles in developed nations. In the U.S. the need for strong soldiers during World War II prompted advances in technology and transportation. Innovative ways to stretch the shelf life of foods, reduce waste, and feed more people were of utmost importance. Much was uncertain in times of war, but food security for soldiers was important in the effort to win the war. The sudden demand for convenience and increased shelf life of foods resulted in a gold rush-like era, prompting marketers and food manufacturers to espouse the benefits of new processed food products.

The mass market welcomed the newfound convenience of processed foods as it enhanced freedom of lifestyle and allowed for more free time away from the daily, often daunting, task of cooking meals. It was not all about convenience though. People loved processed foods, many of which had smoother textures, longer shelf lives; food companies seduced us with plenty of saltier and sweeter products to explore and indulge in. This redirection towards food processing and shift in the dietary staples of the nation is significant. We should recognize the health effects of processed foods and the need to reduce consumption to promote healthy weight, sustained weight loss, and mental well-being.

Fast forward a few decades to the late 1970s and early 1980s, and the food industry has taken food processing to a new level. Government subsidies supported mass production of staple grains like corn, wheat, and soy. These key crops grown in abundance were then used to produce a great number of heavily processed commercial food ingredients used in an endless array of highly processed food products that by and large lack vitamins, minerals, fiber, antioxidants, and other natural substances we need for good health.

Not only were processed foods widely available with many options, but by the mid-eighties, the public was learning a new dietary language of health-related terms due to major food companies' marketing efforts. Much of the discussion and concerns about food now centered around terms like fiber, carbohydrates, amino acids, monounsaturated fats, polyunsaturated fats, antioxidants, probiotics, and polyphenols, just to name a few. In one regard, our understanding of human nutrition was greatly advancing in the latter half of the twentieth century. Product labels required by the Food and Drug Administration (FDA) allowed consumers to compare the nutritional values of products with Recommended Daily Allowances (RDAs) determined by the Institute of Medicine's Food and Nutrition Board.[4] Yet as a nation, we were becoming more distracted and confused about a healthy diet. We were losing sight of traditional diets and what constitutes a basic healthy diet. Or perhaps we were losing sight of what's more important than the quantity or number of calories, and that's the quality of calories and overall balance and pattern of the foods we eat on a regular basis. The common reductionist way of evaluating the healthfulness of individual foods as "good" or "bad" is not only misleading but also confuses our understanding of what we all can agree are basic health food staples.

HEALTH OF A NATION: MENTAL HEALTH

There's no better time than now to increase our focus on the importance of addressing mental health disorders. Per year, it's estimated that nearly 1 out of 5 Americans (or approximately 43.8 million) will experience mental illness.[5] Furthermore, over 10 million people in the U.S. are living with a serious mental illness, which impairs daily functions and significantly impedes major life activities.[6] Approximately 18%

of American adults live with an anxiety disorder and nearly 7% of American adults live with major depression.[7]

Throughout much of history, depression and mental health concerns were mostly considered as the result of supernatural forces or imbalances of "humors", which according to ancient Greek and Roman physicians were bodily fluids that needed to be in balance in order to promote good health.[8] In the early 20th century, mental illness, such as depression, was thought by many to result from deficiencies in character or resilience, or even from an impoverished upbringing. Mental illness in this era was therefore often mischaracterized and dealt with by trying to rid the afflicted from "evil spirits." However, since advancing our scientific understanding of biological psychiatry in the latter part of the 20th century, the predominant theory suggests that the proper treatment for depression is a combination of psychotherapy and counseling, as needed, along with different antidepressant drugs to correct imbalances of neurotransmitters in the brain.

In the last half-century or so, advancements in science resulted in an exponential increase in our understanding of the brain and mental health. The current, prevailing theory that an imbalance of neurotransmitters — and the pharmaceutical regulation of this imbalance — is now challenged by some health experts (especially integrative and functional medicine practitioners) as short-sighted and only a piece of the puzzle in treating depression and other mental health disorders. Relatively newfound in the West (health practitioners in the Eastern hemisphere have been espousing such healthy diet and lifestyle habits for centuries), a more holistic understanding of mental illness along with advancements in science allows us to better determine what constitutes an optimal dietary intake for mental well-being.

We now understand that besides basic physical needs such as adequate water, food, shelter, clean air, and hydration, human beings also have basic psychological needs that should be met to promote more joyful and fulfilling lives. These lifestyle factors make an important contribution to mental health and are recognized from a more holistic perspective of health, but may not be recognized in the traditional practice of medicine and psychiatry in the U.S. today.

As technology has dramatically expanded our ability to study the health and function of the brain and gut, our continuously evolving understanding of the link between gut health and brain health is likely to revolutionize modern health care. In the following chapters, we will explore this link in detail. A common barrier to improving poor gut health (for many, not all, people with mental illness) must be addressed strategically before adopting a general healthful diet that promotes mental well-being. For many people without any sort of chronic or acute gastrointestinal problems, such as irritable bowel syndrome (IBS) or inflammatory bowel diseases (IBD), a healthful eating pattern can be implemented immediately or gradually. However, for somebody living with IBS or IBD (not limited to), there needs to be a strategy to improve gastrointestinal problems before advancing to an overall healthy eating pattern (discussed in Chapter 4).

High Stress + Lack of Self-Care + Poor Diet = Recipe for Disaster

There's no doubt that the pace of life for most people in our time seems fast and for most of us, this means increased stress. With so many distractions to encounter daily — instant news, smartphone notifications, text messages, emails, and advertisements, just to name a few — it's no wonder that these distractions tend to promote stress for many people. Although some stress is normal and even healthy in some instances, when you live in a chronic state of stress, this affects your digestive function and consequently can impact your mood. It may also decrease your ability to cope with stress, eventually increasing the risk of worse harm to both physical and mental health.

The food choices you make on a daily basis may be compounding the effects of your daily stressors. Keep in mind that chronic stress is related to chronic inflammation. In other words, your diet choices can help to extinguish the fires of chronic inflammation or they can stoke the flames of chronic inflammation. As you'll learn in Chapter 2, chronic inflammation can contribute to serious health problems when left unmanaged. Chronic stress and inflammation are strongly linked with poor mental health and so we must recognize this link before improving mental health through lifestyle changes.

From everyday life stressors to major life-event or even occasional traumatic experiences, everybody deals with stressors throughout the course of life. One important question to consider is how well you manage everyday stressors. This is what "self-care" is all about. Self-care is very important for managing your everyday stressors. Adequate sleep, physical activity, and other self-care measures, such as advancing health knowledge, practicing good hygiene, and of course, eating a nutritious diet, all have a major impact on your ability to cope with stress. Those who do not manage stress very well are more likely to suffer from anxiety, depression, or other mental health disorders.

One of the most expensive health problems and leading causes of disability in the world today is depression, affecting approximately 350 million people worldwide. This costs the U.S. an estimated $100 billion each year. Over 48,000 people committed suicide in 2018.[9] Although medications for depression, anxiety, and other mental health diagnoses are helpful and even life-saving for many people, unfortunately, some estimates suggest the majority of people either do not notice benefit from treatment or are only partially helped with their condition.[10] It's also important to note there are many unpleasant side effects that often result from taking different medications for mental health disorders. Even more concerning is that because of these side effects, sometimes people end up not properly taking their medications. These common side effects are not limited to but can range from weight gain to nausea to sexual dysfunction and even impairment in cognition or mood. Furthermore, some depression medications, when taken for long periods of time or against doctors' orders can have the opposite of intended effect and induce more depression or make it difficult to get off these medications without other undesirable effects, especially if abruptly stopped. The point here is that medications all too often are but one piece of improving mental health outcomes and unfortunately have common negative side effects for some.

For many people, lifestyle changes are arguably just as important (or perhaps even more important) as taking medications for improving mental health. Although you might have a higher likelihood of major depression or other common mental health conditions due to the genes you inherit from your parents — or resulting from factors outside of your control such as trauma or problems in utero — the lifestyle factors discussed in this book play a profound role in helping manage troublesome symptoms and help to enhance the quality of life for those with depression and/or anxiety. This more holistic perspective of health (and mental health in particular) discussed in this book unfortunately still hasn't been widely accepted in mainstream American culture. However, this sentiment is slowly changing as we can no longer ignore the power of an optimal diet and healthy lifestyle for the health of the brain and the health of the "second brain" (discussed in Chapters 3 and 4).

ONE IMPORTANT NOTE:

It's important that you understand depression, anxiety, and other mental health diagnoses are very complex health problems. I am not here to tell you that what you eat is simply THE cause or cure for any health problem. However, I am writing this book to help inform you that what you eat on a daily basis — besides other lifestyle factors also discussed — greatly impacts not only your physical health but also your gut health and may affect your mood and serve as one more effective tool in your toolbox of resources to manage depression and anxiety. In other words, your daily food choices and behaviors are a significant piece of the puzzle for helping you feel the best you can, along with other models of treatment that can help, such as working with a therapist, and/or with a psychiatrist for medications.

PART I

MENTAL WELL-BEING & FOOD-MOOD CONNECTION

One cannot think well, love well, sleep well, if one has not dined well.

VIRGINIA WOOLF

CHAPTER 1

ANXIETY, DEPRESSION, AND OTHER MENTAL HEALTH DISORDERS

THE FOOD-MOOD CONNECTION

Human beings are amazingly complicated. Our behaviors and moods can be influenced by so many different factors. We experience an extensive array of emotions, come from varied backgrounds with a wide array of adverse childhood experiences and traumas, all of which may contribute to anxiety, depression, and other mental health disorders. We have diverse skills and abilities that are important to consider when adopting healthy lifestyle changes to improve mental well-being. Human beings are very resilient and with the right treatment plan, lifestyle changes, and support system, have an impressive ability to overcome and improve symptoms of anxiety, depression, or other mental health disorders.

What you eat is so important that for some people, healthy diet changes alone have the potential to be effective to improve mood and energy levels. This may be especially helpful for those with few or no adverse childhood experiences, or other factors related to depression and anxiety, but still experience low energy and occasional depressed moods. Even if you are aware of non-dietary reasons that contribute to anxiety or depression, optimizing your dietary intake can give you more energy, improve your mood, and strengthen your immune system to better fight off infections, and overall may improve your sense of mental well-being.

In recent years, many people are realizing that what they eat has a direct impact on their physical health. However, not as many people realize (they may perhaps ignore) the impact that food choices and nutrition can have on their mood, energy level, and overall mental health. In fact, eating a nutrient-depleted diet, such as the "standard American diet", is more likely to affect your mood, stamina, irritability, and ability to concentrate much sooner than it will affect the health of your eyes, heart, or bones. This is your day-to-day health and brain health is especially dependent upon a steady supply of nutrients. How you feel in the afternoon is partially dependent on the nutrients you eat or don't eat in the morning. Your mood and energy level in the evening is partially dependent on what you eat or don't eat at breakfast, lunch, and dinner. Similarly, sleep quality and how you feel in the morning is somewhat dependent on what you eat the few hours before bedtime.

It's not just the food choices that are important, adequate hydration is one of the most basic, cheap, and simple steps you can do to promote good health. Hydration is important for too many reasons to discuss here. With regard to promoting a positive mood, we already discussed the importance of getting plenty of nutrient-rich whole foods in the diet. Well, all these important vitamins and minerals need water to help carry and deliver these nutrients to all the working cells in the body and the brain. Excessive alcohol or large daily doses of caffeine from coffee, soda, energy drinks may also be another important behavior to modify in order to find greater results from other diet changes. This is particularly important for those with sleep problems along with mental health problems. Too much alcohol or caffeine not only contributes to dehydration and depletion of important nutrients in the body, but it can also affect your sleep quality. So be aware of how your usual intake of fluids affects your hydration and sleep.

COMMON MENTAL HEALTH DISORDERS LINKED WITH DIET

Although there are over 250 different mental health disorders (according to the DSM-5), I'll mention some of the more common and well-known conditions that are linked with diet. Keep in mind that nutrition for mental health disorders is still a relatively new specialty of nutrition science and so there are still many questions left unsettled. However, this doesn't mean we shouldn't discuss all the potential improvements to many of these mental health disorders that may be achieved through diet and lifestyle changes. Among other developing areas of science, the emerging specialties of neuropsychiatry, nutrigenomics, and metabolomics will help us answer many questions in the years to come. Perhaps these fields of science may even lay the groundwork for future improvements in psychiatry and mental health outcomes.

Mood disorders: depression and bipolar disorder

One of the more established links between nutrition and mental health is that of the essential fatty acids called omega-3 fats and different types of depression and bipolar disorders. We cannot say yet that by simply increasing intake of omega-3 fats we will effectively treat or improve depression. It can be said with a little more certainty that by increasing intake of omega-3 fats in those who are deficient, it is likely to help improve outcomes of current treatments or improve symptoms of major depression or bipolar disorder.[1] However, there are still some inconsistencies found in research about how effective this can be. Part of the explanation for inconsistent findings among studies likely depends on the severity of the depression of those included in the study and the total amount and relative amounts of different types of omega-3 fatty acids used in various studies. Research suggests that it's the EPA type of omega-3 (rather than DHA) that is more important and offers the beneficial anti-inflammatory and, therefore, antidepressant effects desired. It may be the EPA type of omega-3 that future studies need to focus on as we learn more about the potential benefits of increasing intake of omega-3 fats, whether through foods or a dietary supplement.

Anxiety-related disorders

One less researched and understood link is that between anxiety-related disorders and diet. Nonetheless, this link has the potential to be further explored and explained. Despite limited conclusive evidence in science on diet and anxiety, don't underestimate the power of a healthful, balanced diet to control levels of anxiety. In clinical practice, I often hear people explain how much better they feel after significant diet changes, not only with regard to more stable energy levels throughout the day, but also regarding their ability to relax and not feel quite as stressed continuing to face normal day to day stressors and responsibilities. The link between diet and anxiety is mostly explained through a few different mechanisms.

First, we need a steady supply of certain vitamins, minerals, and amino acids in the diet for the body to produce neurotransmitters that regulate mood and sleep, and help us relax. Furthermore, certain strains of gut bugs help to produce serotonin, GABA, dopamine, and acetylcholine within the digestive tract.[2] These are key neurotransmitters that contribute to mood and relaxation, and help regulate sleep schedules.

Secondly, the lack of stable blood sugar control (abrupt spikes followed by rapid drops in blood sugar) is also likely to impact one's sense of relaxation or anxiety levels. This is discussed more in the next section, *Wholesome Foods Promote Healthy Moods*. Lastly, an unbalanced microbiome is likely to promote a state of chronic inflammation, along with a disruption in the signaling systems involved in regulating stress hormones. Overall, this state of gut dysbiosis signals from the second brain to the main brain, a state of unease and distress. On the other hand, as stated in *The Anti-Anxiety Diet*, a balanced and "symbiotic gut drives a happy, mellow mind."[3] Perhaps it is this chronic disruption of a normal functioning digestive tract accompanied by a diet low in nutrients that is experienced as a sense of anxiety.

Don't forget to think about what you're drinking. Excessive intake of alcohol or caffeine may impact your normal regulation of neurotransmitters and contribute to a sense of anxiety or anxiety-related disorders. Although small amounts of alcohol might help some people feel relaxed, with time, or with too much alcohol, this can also impact the regulation of your neurotransmitters and consequently contribute to anxiety in the long run, more than it helps. Caffeine works by inhibiting the release of the calming neurotransmitter GABA in the brain. So, first and foremost, drink plenty of water or other non-caffeinated beverages, and limit the total amount of alcohol or caffeine you drink. For people who have a history of alcoholism or are notably sensitive to caffeine, it is probably best to abstain from alcoholic or caffeinated drinks.

Schizophrenia and related psychotic disorders

A more complex or troublesome group of mental health disorders includes schizophrenia and related psychotic disorders. According to the American Psychiatric Association, "schizophrenia is characterized by delusions, hallucinations, disorganized speech and behavior, and other symptoms that cause social or occupational dysfunction."[4] Thankfully, our understanding of these mental illnesses has evolved over the years and researchers are taking a more open-minded, closer look at the role of diet in these disorders. Among many other factors that contribute to these complex mental illnesses, a low-quality diet without adequate intakes of fruits, vegetables, whole grains, and other fibrous foods is a common link found in mental health disorders.[5] Researchers at King's College London compiled the results from 31 different studies on this topic and found that people who had schizophrenia were more likely to have higher intakes of calories and processed foods that provide unhealthy amounts of saturated fats, salt, and refined sugars.[6]

Consider how a nutritionally poor diet can contribute to metabolic dysfunction and chronic inflammation. People who have schizophrenia may be at higher risk of problems from this dysfunction and inflammation given that they tend to have lower levels of essential fatty acids, higher levels of pro-inflammatory compounds (cytokines) in the blood when tested, and they're more likely to have increased oxidative stress. Overall, this can have a detrimental effect on the normal functioning of the metabolism and may even disrupt the production and regulation of neurotransmitters. Although the exact cause of schizophrenia and other psychotic disorders is not well understood, leading researchers suggest that it's a dysregulation of dopamine and other neurotransmitters that is mostly responsible for the troublesome symptoms seen among people who have these disorders.[7]

Besides the nutrient-depleted diet commonly found in the population, factors such as poor nutrient absorption, excessive alcohol intake, or too much of certain medications can also make these problems more likely. Did you know that when certain vitamin deficiencies are left uncorrected over time, symptoms can get so bad that they can even manifest as psychosis? To be clear, psychosis is not a specific mental illness, rather it is a symptom that is related to a variety of different disorders. It's characterized by "the loss of contact with reality" and can appear in different ways such as "severe confusional state, delusions, hallucinations, and marked impairment in judgment and reasoning."[8] Thus, psychosis can be caused by a variety of factors, such as different medical conditions or even certain nutrient deficiencies. Specifically, deficiencies of B-vitamins such as B-1 (thiamin) or B-3 (niacin), can result in psychotic symptoms. Other B-vitamins — B-6, B-9 (folic acid), and B-12 — are less well understood regarding the cause of these mental illnesses, yet are still critical for neurological health and in some cases may partially explain the causes of psychosis-related disorders.[9]

Also noteworthy, research has shown that supplementation of B-vitamins (such as folate) can improve troubling symptoms.[10] It may be a far stretch to say that inadequate nutrition causes these complex mental health disorders in most cases, but it is safer to say that a nutritious and balanced diet — and possibly even some dietary supplements in certain cases — can reduce the likelihood of experiencing troublesome symptoms of psychotic disorders.

WHOLESOME FOODS PROMOTE HEALTHY MOODS

The word wholesome is a bit vague and could be misleading when used in marketing to suggest the healthfulness of processed food products, so let's be clear on what's meant here. With few exceptions, foods tend to be healthier in their whole, minimally or unprocessed state. For example, a whole apple is healthier (more nutrient-dense, packed with phytonutrients and fiber) than applesauce, and similarly, applesauce is slightly healthier than apple juice. I emphasize the importance of including more of the "good" foods rather than simply avoiding the "bad" foods as many people tend to label foods and mistakenly oversimplify this matter.

Because we are not perfect beings, we should not be aiming for a perfect diet. In my opinion, there's no such thing. Besides, more popular and rigid types of diets are often limited, become boring, and can easily result in lost interest in eating. So when it comes to eating wholesome foods, one might not aim to avoid all processed foods, rather to focus on eating minimally-processed and whole foods most of the time or as often as possible, and to either avoid or eat few foods that are highly-processed. If you must, have these highly processed food products sparingly as an exception to your daily food choices. It's important to note that everybody makes changes at their own pace and so we'll discuss later in the book about how to eat more wholesome foods and how to find your best approach to sustainable, lifestyle changes to ultimately improve your mood and overall mental well-being.

One of the leaders on the subject of nutrition for mental health, Leslie Korn, put it simply: "Mood follows food, and mood swings follow blood sugar swings."[11] This is especially true for those who drink a lot of sugar-sweetened beverages (soda, juices, energy drinks, etc.) and eat a lot of food products high in refined grains, such as white flours, and added sugars. These food products are typically consumed in large quantities in the "standard American diet". When you eat a lot of these processed foods that lack fiber, healthy fats, and protein, this produces a rapid rise in blood sugar (blood glucose) which can result in a short-lived feeling or burst of energy and feeling good. However, the body must then compensate for this spike in blood glucose by releasing a surge of insulin (except for a person with type 1 diabetes whose pancreas no longer produces insulin). Over the next few hours, this relatively abrupt release of insulin can result in low energy, increased appetite, and low blood sugars. Not to mention the fat storage also promoted by high levels of insulin.

This scenario of blood sugar dysregulation is more likely to occur following an inconsistent meal pattern or a lack of balance of macronutrients for long periods — in other words, when you are not getting adequate protein, fiber, or fat to slow the digestion of high loads of carbohydrates frequently consumed at meals and snacks. In more severe cases, an unbalanced diet and inconsistent meal pattern can promote what is called reactive hypoglycemia. These unstable fluctuations of blood sugar sometimes have dangerous effects and are likely to have a direct impact on day-to-day mood and energy levels. In many cases, this daily roller coaster ride of blood sugar levels can easily be corrected through following a balanced diet and not skipping meals, which we will discuss in Part III.

Remember the importance of balance and try not to skip your breakfast, lunch, or dinner. It's okay if once in a while you get too busy and must skip a meal, or perhaps you're following an informed intermittent fasting practice, but don't allow this to be your normal daily habit. For those trying to lose weight or better manage blood sugar levels, if you have longer than four to five hours between meals, plan to have a balanced snack.

Unlike refined grains and added sugars, whole grains are wholesome and more fulfilling since they're packed with essential vitamins, minerals, fiber, and even provide some essential fats and protein. This better balance of macronutrients in whole grains produces a different, longer-lasting stabilizing effect on the blood sugar, and greater satiety (sense of fullness). Of all of the grain-based foods that you eat (including bread, pasta, cereal, tortillas, rice, pastries, etc.) at least half of them should be whole grains. I personally would argue this is a modest recommendation. For optimal health, perhaps we should be eating far less than 50% of products made from refined grains. With few exceptions for certain people—such as gluten-containing grains for those with celiac disease or following an elimination trial, or for those following a low-fiber diet—whole grains are nutrient-dense food staples and are a part of most healthy dietary patterns.

Although we must not discount the importance of a well-balanced diet by focusing too much on individual nutrients, it's valuable to know the role some of these nutrients serve for mental well-being. Note that when key nutrients are lacking in the diet, a nutrient deficiency alone may have harmful effects on mood. In certain cases, deficiencies of various nutrients are potentially a key causative factor in a variety of different mental illnesses. Moreover, the "standard American diet" lacks fruits, vegetables, and whole grains which likely results in widespread deficient intakes of critical nutrients, such as essential fatty acids, minerals, and B-vitamins.[12]

KEY NUTRIENTS LINKED WITH MENTAL HEALTH

Essential fatty acids (EFAs)

Besides the protective and energy-providing roles of dietary fats, a certain type of polyunsaturated essential fats — omega-3 fatty acids — have been recently suggested as a complementary mode of treatment (taken with other treatments) for depression. Again, note the word "essential" because without adequate intake of certain types of fats, humans will die and so the importance can hardly be overstated here. This is particularly true when we're talking about brain health. Inadequate levels of EFAs (particularly omega-3 fats) are linked with quite a variety of mental health disorders, such as depression, bipolar disorder, attention deficit and attention deficit hyperactivity disorders (ADD/ADHD), anxiety-related disorders, and even schizophrenia and other psychotic disorders. However, given the relatively inconsistent or weak links among some of these, let's briefly focus more on the role of omega-3 fats on depressive disorders. Compared to the relatively limited or inconclusive evidence for using omega-3 fats to improve outcomes for the other neurologic conditions, this is one common and more strongly supported link. So strong that we can even begin to talk about inadequate intakes of omega-3 fats being a potential cause for depression rather than simply a link found in research.

One impressive study from 2014 compiled the results of 19 randomized clinical trials that looked at the relationship between omega-3 supplementation and depressive symptoms in different populations of people with a diagnosis of depressive disorder or without a clinical diagnosis, but having depressive symptoms. This study, published more recently, concluded that omega-3 supplementation resulted in significant clinical benefits in symptoms of depression.[13] However, other studies in the past have reported less impressive results, such as finding no significant benefit in depressive symptoms compared to a placebo. In 2012, another similar study compiled the results of 13 randomized, placebo-controlled clinical trials studying the effectiveness of omega-3 supplementation on depressive symptoms and failed to find any significant effect.[14] This 2012 study also researched the reasons why these different clinical trials often result in different conclusions and found a variety of reasons that contribute to the inconsistency of results. For example, shorter durations of trials and whether or not people with other mental illnesses were included in the studies are both factors that can influence the results of such studies. Long story short, the potential of omega-3 fatty acids for treating a variety of different mental health conditions — particularly depression — is only barely beginning to be realized.

ESSENTIAL MINERALS AND VITAMINS

Magnesium

Magnesium is an essential mineral we must get from the diet, required for an impressive variety of physiological processes and biochemical reactions in the body. Similar to essential fatty acids, it's importance can hardly be overstated. Magnesium is important for the nervous system and brain function because it acts as a common coenzyme (activator of chemical reactions in the body) for more than 300 unique enzymatic processes. This is critical to support smooth and efficient communication between the central nervous system and brain. In turn, adequate magnesium intake — most Americans don't get enough — may promote a more relaxed, improved sense of mental well-being.

Furthermore, magnesium deficiency is known to contribute to various neurological disorders and so without adequate magnesium for the nerve cells to function effectively, this can contribute to neuronal disturbances, which may ultimately promote a sense of depression, anxiety, or even attention deficit disorder among other conditions.

There's also research demonstrating that these neuronal deficiencies are not only influenced by inadequate dietary intake of magnesium but also from stress hormones or excessive calcium intake.[15] This is interesting considering that many Americans live in a chronic state of stress, don't eat enough magnesium-rich foods, while usual calcium intake levels tend to vary considerably between different populations, age groups, and gender.[16] Research suggests that when someone has neuronal deficiencies of magnesium, they are likely to respond positively to increased magnesium intake. One might then infer that those who have chronic low dietary intakes of magnesium and high levels of stress could benefit from taking a magnesium supplement or, perhaps better yet, benefit by including magnesium-rich foods at most meals.

Though it's well known that magnesium is critical for neurological health and overall brain health, the mechanisms for which this essential mineral impacts symptoms of depression, anxiety, or other mental health conditions are not well understood. With the available research, we can't determine a cause-and-effect relationship between magnesium intake and depression or anxiety. However, there are several studies that have found an inverse relationship between magnesium intake and symptoms of depression.[17,18,19,20] In other words, these studies found that those who ate less magnesium were more likely to be depressed.

Magnesium can be abundantly provided in the diet by eating a good variety of vegetables, nuts, seeds, whole grains, legumes, and lean meats. Some of the best sources tend to come from various darker colored plant-based foods such as spinach, quinoa, black beans, edamame, almonds, and whole wheat products, just to name a few. Similar to fiber, the amount of magnesium can also be affected by the degree of food processing. For example, an average slice of white bread only has about one third or one quarter the magnesium content you'll find in a comparable slice of whole-grain bread.

Zinc

Similar to how important magnesium is for speeding up chemical processes in the body, zinc is another essential mineral that is necessary for over 100 unique enzymatic processes.[21] From a mental health perspective, zinc is arguably one of the most important "trace minerals" (needed in very small quantities) because it has multiple functions, including stress management and maintaining proper immune system response. Although the exact mechanisms are not well understood, the relationship between low blood levels of zinc and depression may be explained through the balancing role it plays in maintaining normal management of hormones, neurotransmitters, and the development and regeneration of the nervous system cells.[22]

Although red meats, dairy, and poultry tend to be the main sources of zinc in most Americans' diets, per serving, no food provides more zinc than oysters. Just about two to three ounces of oysters can provide up to two to four times the recommended dietary allowance (RDA) of zinc for most adults. Otherwise, good sources include legumes such as beans, lentils and peas, nuts and seeds, whole grains, and fortified breakfast cereals.

Selenium

Similar to magnesium and zinc, selenium is an essential mineral that is important for maintaining proper regulation of hormones and neurotransmitters. Selenium also acts as an antioxidant and protects against cellular damage and inflammation. Similar to the other essential minerals, the exact mechanisms of how levels of selenium might affect mood or symptoms of depression are not well understood. However, one thing that research is clear about is the importance of having adequate intakes of this micronutrient for maintaining the normal function of the nervous system, and brain health in general.

B-vitamins and iron

B-vitamins and iron are included together here because of the similar symptoms that can result from some of these deficiencies and can sometimes be mistaken for one another. In Table 1 below, you will see a summary of the most relevant B-vitamins as well as iron. Though not all of them are included in the table below, there are eight different B-vitamins that are grouped together because of their similar functions in helping the body metabolize and provide energy from carbohydrates and fats, and breaking down the proteins in the foods you eat. Similar to the roles that magnesium, zinc, and selenium serve in speeding up biochemical reactions, B-vitamins are important helpers to enzymes that enable chemical reactions to occur seamlessly. We also need B-vitamins and iron for blood to serve its role in delivering oxygen to the body's working cells. B-vitamins are not only critical for a normal functioning nervous system, but also for maintaining a healthy metabolism and accessing the energy in the foods we eat.

Eventually, deficiencies of certain B-vitamins can get so bad that psychosis may develop. So, the importance of B-vitamins for overall brain and mental health can hardly be overstated. Although deficiencies of some B-vitamins tend to be rare in developed areas of the world, there's a variety of different factors that impact the body's ability to absorb these important nutrients even when good dietary sources are eaten regularly. Note that excess caffeine can increase how much of these nutrients are released from the body and lost in the urine. Most food sources of B-vitamins tend to have a variety of B-vitamins. This circles back to the importance of eating a balanced and varied diet rather than artificially supplementing these nutrients. However, there are certain cases where someone may benefit from taking dietary supplements and we'll revisit this in Chapter 5.

TABLE 1. Iron and B-vitamins: deficiency symptoms, food sources, and populations at higher risk

Nutrient	Deficiency symptoms/syndrome	Food sources (not limited to)	Conditions and/or those at higher risk
Iron	Anemia; difficulty concentrating, fatigue, weakness, decreased immune function and regulation of body temperature *Although deficiency more common, excess iron can also be a problem*	Meat, seafood, nuts, beans, fortified grain products, some vegetables	Pregnancy, infants/ young children, certain inflammatory gastrointestinal (GI) disorders, frequent blood donors, or women with heavy menstruation
B-3 - Niacin	Confusion, fatigue, and pellagra ("The 4 D's"- dermatitis, diarrhea, dementia, and eventually death)	Tuna, salmon, beef liver, beef, chicken breast, beef, mushrooms, turkey, brown rice, avocado, and peanuts	Alcoholism, malabsorptive conditions
Biotin	Nausea, anorexia, dry scaly dermatitis, depression *deficiency very rare*	Organ meats, beef liver, fish, eggs, nuts, seeds, sweet potatoes	Alcoholism, malabsorptive conditions
B-6	Dermatitis, glossitis (tongue inflammation), confusion, depression *deficiency is uncommon*	Fish, organ meats, fortified breakfast cereals, poultry, bananas, potatoes	Elderly, alcoholism, use of certain medications, those with impaired kidney function, certain autoimmune disorders and other malabsorptive conditions
Folate (B-9)	Anemia; confusion, depression, diarrhea, fatigue	Dark leafy green vegetables, spinach, asparagus, lima beans, edamame, avocado, kidney beans	Alcoholism; malabsorptive conditions, use of certain medications
B-12	Anemia; confusion, depression, fatigue, weakness, constipation, loss of appetite, glossitis	Fish, meat, poultry, eggs, milk, and milk products	Elderly, alcoholism, malabsorptive conditions, vegetarians/ vegans, and after certain GI surgeries

WORKING TOWARDS GUIDELINES

Unlike diabetes, heart disease, kidney disease, high blood pressure, or a variety of other medical conditions, there are no specific dietary guidelines to follow for optimal mental health. Although we may not understand the link between diet and individual mental health conditions quite as clearly as we do for other chronic illnesses, the answers about what is the best diet — or at least what are the most important dietary factors — for promoting optimal well-being are becoming increasingly apparent in recent years. We may not have clearly established guidelines, though the consensus is emerging among researchers, even among those experts with contrasting opinions about what constitutes the healthiest diet. Thanks to devoted Ph.D. researchers, medical doctors, and other pioneers in this field, such as Leslie Korn, Martha Clare Morris, Frank Sacks, Felice Jacka, Ruth Leyse-Wallace, and Gerard Mullin among many others, a path has been paved for establishing more specific dietary guidelines for mental health.

Furthermore, the discussion of nutrition for mental health is not limited to the various nutrients discussed above. There are other nutrients with less understood links to mental health. There are also different food components, such as antioxidants and other phytonutrients. The synergistic effects of these we frankly have not researched sufficiently and, therefore, we don't fully understand the potential impact on the brain and mental health. So, until we have more clearly established guidelines, we can focus on what most of the leading experts can agree on and use model dietary patterns accordingly.

CHAPTER 2

CHRONIC INFLAMMATION: ARE YOU FUELING THE FIRE OF DEPRESSION?

Whenyou think about the word *fire*, what other thoughts first come to mind? Perhaps they are negative thoughts about a bad past episode of getting burned or maybe even a disastrous loss from a fire that you or a loved one experienced. Or maybe your first thought might be more positive, bringing back dear memories of telling ghost stories and making shish kebabs or s'mores with family by a campfire, or how the warmth of the fireplace keeps you comfortable in the winter. Whatever your thoughts about fire, note that fire can be either very purposeful and even life-saving, or it can be harmful and destructive.

Similar to fire in this regard, inflammation in the body can either be helpful and even life-saving — for example, by preventing the spread of infection — or it can contribute to pain and cause harm to your body and increase your chances of getting a variety of chronic illnesses that are associated with chronic inflammation. Some of these also happen to be the biggest killers in the U.S., such as heart disease, diabetes, Alzheimer's disease, and even cancer.[1] Diseases related to systemic chronic inflammation are the most significant cause of death in the world today.[2]

To understand the link between inflammation and depression, we must first discuss the characteristics of clinical depression and note the similarity of clinical signs and symptoms in inflammation and depressive disorders. These commonalities should not be overlooked when treating depression, as this speaks directly to the importance of a healthy diet and lifestyle. In short, combating chronic inflammation enhances treatments for depression, such as therapy and/or medications. It's unfortunately common for depression to be inadequately controlled by medications. One study found a significant link in those with higher levels of inflammatory markers and resistance to conventional antidepressant treatments.[3] This suggests the potential of an anti-inflammatory diet to enhance the effectiveness of current antidepressant medications.

Moreover, people with various other inflammatory conditions also suffer from similar signs and symptoms common to sufferers of clinical depression. For example, chronic autoimmune diseases, or more acute conditions among those receiving certain medical treatments (e.g., interferon therapy for hepatitis C and certain forms of cancer) tend to have notably higher levels of inflammatory markers in the body. Elevated levels of inflammatory markers in the blood are even found in those who have clinical depression but are otherwise considered in good physical health.[4]

Besides some of the complex scientific details discussed briefly in this chapter, the important thing to understand is that everyday lifestyle choices — including what you eat, your level of physical activity, how well you manage everyday stress, how much quality sleep you get, and even your daily exposure to environmental toxins — all play a role in controlling the fires of chronic inflammation. Therefore, your everyday lifestyle choices may be either fueling the fires of inflammation and, consequently your signs and symptoms of depression, or they may be helping to extinguish the fire of chronic inflammation and depression.

ACUTE OR CHRONIC: A GOOD THING GONE BAD?

Let's pause to understand what inflammation is because this normal process in the body is not always a bad thing and is very important to your health. In fact, when the body triggers an inflammatory state, this is just a natural way of signaling to the immune system that the body has encountered an injury or an "invader." More specifically, the detection occurs in the blood. For example, when you cut your finger, you will first notice the sensation of pain and you may bleed; but shortly thereafter, you will notice the cut begins to get red and swollen. The change in color and swelling is due to the body signaling the immune system to react by sending different types of white blood cells to the injured tissue, thereby protecting you from any infection spreading inside the body and creating more health problems. In other words, inflammation is a natural process of the immune system, protecting from further invasion or irritation of the skin tissue and, ultimately, helping overcome any infections that could even be deadly. This is an example of *acute* inflammation that occurs because of the injured tissue. Other potential causes of acute inflammation may occur from infections with various bacteria, parasites, or fungi.

Unlike the necessary protection of the body's natural fighting mechanism that occurs from situations like an infection or the finger cut or other similar injuries, when the body is in a *chronic* state of inflammation — largely the result of lifestyle factors (discussed in the Afterword) — there is a higher likelihood of developing a variety of different chronic diseases. Specifically, some of the biggest killers of most Americans such as diabetes, cardiovascular diseases, and chronic obstructive pulmonary disease (COPD) are linked with inflammation. The link between inflammation and chronic illness does not stop there. Other diseases linked with chronic inflammation include cancer, Alzheimer's disease, allergies, arthritis, and other joint diseases[5] just to name a few others. Even obesity is linked with chronic inflammation!

This means that through your daily lifestyle choices, you can either fuel the fires of inflammation (for example, eat a pro-inflammatory "standard American diet" and have a sedentary lifestyle) or you can take control of your health and calm the fires of chronic inflammation and, ultimately, help your body prevent these various chronic diseases from developing. If you already suffer from a chronic inflammatory condition, you can make healthy changes, and eventually, you might notice improvements in pain and/or depression.

Take this information with a word of caution. Not everybody with major depression is necessarily in a state of chronic inflammation. Furthermore, it may not be likely in standard clinical practice to notice if your body has been chronically inflamed, and primary-care providers might not routinely monitor different markers (biomarkers) of inflammation in lab tests. If you suffer from depressive disorder and medications combined with psychotherapy have not helped much in the past, and you are wondering if you're in a state of chronic inflammation, ask your healthcare provider if they can test some of these "inflammatory biomarkers" such as C-reactive protein and various cytokines (interleukin-1, interleukin-6, and tumor necrosis factor).[6]

Besides the clearly established link between inflammation and many chronic diseases mentioned above, the research on the link between chronic inflammation and depressive disorder is a relatively new area of research and reflects our recently advanced understanding of the way in which everyday lifestyle factors are a major contributor to depression. This connection is now largely explained by what some researchers call the "inflammatory theory of depression."[7] Although the exact mechanisms of the role of inflammation on depression are still being researched, chronic inflammation can alter the metabolism of monoamine neurotransmitters, like dopamine and serotonin. This can result in decreased amounts of these important neurotransmitters available for working nerve cells, which is likely to end up promoting a depressed mood.

Let's not forget that depression is a complex disease and can be deeply rooted in or triggered by different circumstances for different people. Addressing adverse childhood experiences and traumas may also factor in effectively treating depression. For some, this could require some extensive therapy. Furthermore, it must be noted that inflammation is not necessary to cause major depression, nor is it sufficient to cause depression in and of itself.[8] However, the important thing to understand is that chronic inflammation may be a contributing factor if you have clinical depression, while the foods that you eat on a daily basis may have either pro-inflammatory or anti-inflammatory effects. In Part III, you will learn more about dietary patterns that are good models to follow because they can have powerful anti-inflammatory effects, help you lose weight, and improve overall mental well-being.

FURTHER EVIDENCE OF THE INFLAMMATION–DEPRESSION LINK

The typical signs and symptoms of clinical depression vary from fatigue, difficulty concentrating, and sleep problems to aches, body pains, and other flu-like symptoms. These common clinical complaints from those who suffer from depressive disorder are also experienced in those who have undergone certain medical treatments, such as interferon therapy for treatment of hepatitis C (not as common today compared to years ago) or certain types of cancer. These concerning "major side effects" can even lead to suicidal thoughts and are considered so serious that doctors often recommend or require that patients seek additional help from a mental health professional while they are undergoing such treatments.[9]

Interferons are a type of signaling protein that signals the body's immune system to fight viruses and other infections, but also causes inflammation. The inflammation-induced adverse effects of such treatments are similar to the symptoms of major depression and, therefore, suggest a link between inflammation and major depression. This apparently strong relationship between mood and inflammation, seen in clinical practice, has prompted focused research, leading to the inflammatory theory of depression. Current research now questions whether inflammation may not only be associated with depression but may actually be one of the causes of depression.

The interferons administered as therapy are a type of inflammatory compound produced in the body called cytokines. Besides the function of cytokines to regulate the immune system, they also affect mood by impacting the production of neurotransmitters such as serotonin, dopamine, and norepinephrine. Let's not forget that it is these three neurotransmitters that the most popular and effective medications used today to treat depression, are designed to modulate. It's not just physical wellness and chronic diseases that can be adversely affected by drugs that induce inflammation, but we now see that mood and overall emotional wellness are likely impacted by chronic inflammation.

PRO-INFLAMMATORY FOODS = STANDARD AMERICAN DIET (SAD)

When doing dietary consults, I'm often asked, "is this food bad for you?" or "is that food good for you?" With such questions, people focus too much on individual foods and do not stop to recognize the more important aspect of food choice, which is the overall pattern of foods you eat throughout the day or throughout your average week. Regarding unhealthy dietary patterns, it is the "standard American diet" that leads the way (and frankly sets the standard) in overindulgence of a variety of foods that promote inflammation and set the stage for many diseases that kill most Americans. "SAD" is a term often used to describe the dietary pattern of many or most Americans who eat too many highly processed foods.

One recent study compared the number of calories and carbohydrates consumed by people eating "ultra-processed foods"— from a variety of foods offered, as much as they would like —to the number of calories and carbohydrates consumed by the same people in a different two-week time period, with the same number of calories and carbohydrates being offered in the foods provided. The study found that in the two-week period where people were offered ultra-processed foods, on average, they ate more than 500 calories extra each day, with over half of the additional calories coming from additional carbohydrates consumed in the diet. Besides eating too much of these foods because they might simply taste good, part of the reason why people overeat these ultra-processed foods is because they tend to lack fiber — a key nutrient we need from foods to feel satisfied after a meal or snack.[10]

Pro-inflammatory foods largely consist of processed food products made mostly with refined grains and sugars and highly refined oils. This SAD diet also includes too much low-quality meat and dairy that contribute to high levels of saturated fats and lack essential fats. Many of these "ultra-processed" food-products and "factory-farmed" meats and dairy tend to include synthetic preservatives, food coloring, hormones, and antibiotics. These common food additives may have unknown consequences that we've yet to discover or fully appreciate from existing research.

Fats: Friend or Foe? Or Both?

Along with carbohydrates and proteins, dietary fats are one of the three macronutrients. A combination of these three macronutrients provides 100% of your caloric intake. Fats (which break down into fatty acids) also provide a rich source of energy or calories, particularly for the brain, which happens to be primarily made up of fats. Dietary fat serves a critical purpose. Some fat serves as a cushion to protect vital organs, keep the body insulated from damage, and protect the lining or membranes of all the cells in the body. Some fat is required in a meal for the absorption of certain nutrients. So there are several reasons why we need fats in the diet. Certain vitamins are fat-soluble which means they can't be absorbed without dietary fats. This group of vitamins include vitamins A, D, E, and K. The outdated advice commonly given in the past to the general public to eat fat-free or low-fat foods is not the best advice nowadays for most people (with few exceptions). The bottom line is that we all need some fats in the diet for health in general, and we need specific types of dietary fats for good mental health in particular.

Different types of dietary fats can have various effects on health. The diverse fats in a particular food is referred to as the "fat profile." Some types of fat can be unhealthy in large amounts yet fine and even have some protective effects in moderation, such as omega-6 polyunsaturated fats and saturated fats; while another type, trans fats are just plain bad for health. There are four different types of fats. But more importantly, there are two different types considered essential for you to eat regularly, with a greater emphasis on one over the other. The essential fats include monounsaturated fats and polyunsaturated fats. The other two types of fats not considered essential for health are saturated fats and trans fats, (hydrogenated oils). Let's take a closer look at each of these.

Saturated fats in most Americans' diets primarily come from a combination of high-fat meat and dairy products, especially from conventionally produced (non-organic) animal-based food products. A few plant-based foods are also high in saturated fats, such as coconuts, palm kernel oil, and palm oil. In the past, we thought saturated fats were more harmful than we now believe they are. This belief was first supported by what is now referred to as the "lipid hypothesis" which suggests that higher intakes of saturated fats and cholesterol cause heart disease.[11] And remember that what is bad for heart health, in general, is also bad for brain health. Although there may be some links between high intakes of saturated fats and cholesterol and likelihood of cardiovascular disease, much of this earlier research that the "lipid hypothesis" was based upon has been questioned owing to the limitations of these research studies. More recent studies have failed to find similar blood cholesterol-increasing effects of saturated fats and cholesterol in foods.[12] Our understanding of nutrition science and the complexities of synergistic effects of eating a balanced, varied diet has greatly evolved. We're now beginning to understand that it's the overall pattern of one's diet that is far more important than the amount of any individual nutrient or a particular food. Stated otherwise, there's plenty of conflicting research available on dietary fats and its link with heart disease over the past several decades. This remains somewhat controversial. For this book however, I must limit the discussion on this and focus on what we all can agree on.

The worst types of fats are trans fats, also referred to as hydrogenated oils. Most of the trans fats in Americans' diets come from highly processed food products, such as deep-fried foods, donuts and other baked goods, just to name a few. Trans fats have no place in a heart- or brain-healthy diet. Such highly processed food products tend to use a lot of cheap, refined oils that not only contribute to inflammation, but also increase risk for heart disease and other health problems. On a more positive note, the Food and Drug Administration ruled in 2015 that trans fats are not safe to eat and as of June 2018, manufacturers in the U.S. are no longer allowed to use these chemically altered fats. It wasn't until January 2021 that the extended compliance deadline for food products in the U.S. market was reached, which meant that any remaining food products made prior to deadline should have worked through the marketplace and no longer be available on store shelves.

Another thing on which health experts agree is the importance of including heart-healthy, essential fats in your daily diet. Regarding the healthy fats, the unsaturated fats are considered essential for good health, hence the name essential fatty acids (EFAs). This includes monounsaturated fats and polyunsaturated fats. In fact, we need them to survive. There is one somewhat confusing rule about which types of fats to emphasize and which to limit. This rule regards what the optimal ratio of one fat to another is. When not eaten in relative balance, too much of certain fats (otherwise, regarded as healthy) can have pro-inflammatory effects while others may have anti-inflammatory effects when eaten in a desirable healthy balance. More specifically, it's the ratio of omega-6 to omega-3 polyunsaturated fats that's believed to be an important factor with regard to inflammation.

One problem is that most Americans tend to get far more than adequate amounts of omega-6 fats — primarily in the form of highly refined oils and grain-fed meats — while not eating nearly enough of the anti-inflammatory omega-3 fatty acids that are more commonly found in fatty fish, leafy greens, nuts and seeds. Bottom line, you shouldn't have to worry about calculating the ideal ratio of different fats or determining exactly how much of each fat you're eating if you generally eat a healthy, balanced dietary pattern (examples in Chapter 7) including a variety of foods with essential fats. Though not all food labels include all of the different types of fats, you can see in Figure 1 below an example of a Nutrition Facts Label that shows the fat profile of avocado oil.

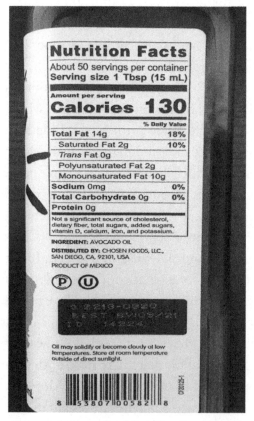

FIGURE 1. Example of Nutrition Facts Label

Given the different "fat profiles" of various foods, be selective about where the fats in your diet are coming from. Unsaturated fats (especially monounsaturated) and omega-3 (one type of polyunsaturated fat) are particularly important for the health of the heart and the brain. Overall, too much unhealthy fat and not enough essential fat could be contributing to chronic inflammation and perhaps contributing to a poor mood. Table 2 below gives examples of pro-inflammatory foods.

TABLE 2. Pro-inflammatory foods and reasons to eat less or avoid*

Pro-Inflammatory Foods - Eat less/Avoid	
Foods	Why eat less/avoid
White bread, bagels, pastries, muffins, crackers, instant rice, high sugar/low fiber cereals, flour-based snack foods, flour tortillas, etc.	High glycemic load- • promotes high fluctuations in blood sugars/insulin levels, may promote inflammation, gut dysbiosis, etc.
Red meats & high-fat dairy products- • conventionally produced, higher in omega-6 fats, lower omega-3s • grass-fed has a healthier fat profile • choose organic if you include dairy Industrial seed oils: • Corn, cottonseed, grapeseed, peanut, safflower, soy, and sunflower oils Deep-fried foods	High in omega-6 fats, saturated and/or trans fats- • although some omega-6 fats are essential, remember most Americans eat far too much of these types of fats, which can promote inflammation • Small amounts of these foods are okay to eat, many Americans eat far too much of these foods
**Dairy, wheat, eggs, artificial flavors, colors and sweeteners (e.g. aspartame) **NOT *necessarily pro-inflammatory to all people, ONLY to those who have a reaction to these foods.*	Common "trigger foods" likely to result in food intolerance and promote IBS-like symptoms (e.g. chronic constipation, diarrhea)

*University of Wisconsin, Department of Family Medicine, Integrative Medicine Patient Handout

ANTI-INFLAMMATORY FOODS

Arguably more important than what Americans eat too much of, a SAD diet lacks enough of the anti-inflammatory foods. Considering the different foods that have anti-inflammatory effects, most of these tend to be limited or even non-existent in many Americans' diets. For example, fatty fish such as salmon, tuna, and sardines. Or extra virgin olive oil, avocados, nuts and seeds. How about dark leafy greens which provide lesser amounts of these essential fats? Certainly, not enough Americans eat enough dark leafy greens. These are all food sources rich in essential fatty acids. If you don't eat any of these on a regular basis, you might want to consider a high-quality omega-3 supplement because this type of fat is so important to eat regularly in your diet for promoting mental well-being. Otherwise, most Americans don't eat enough other nutrient-dense anti-inflammatory staples. Not just dark leafy greens, but think about berries, cruciferous vegetables (e.g. cabbage, cauliflower, kale) or orange, yellow, and red fruits and vegetables. Beyond fruits and veggies, many Americans also don't eat enough beans and other legumes, whole grains and even different spices and herbs. A great variety of these colorful foods have powerful anti-inflammatory effects, so eat them every day, throughout the week, or as often as possible. Table 3 on next page gives examples of anti-inflammatory foods.

FINAL THOUGHTS ON INFLAMMATION

Note that the research on this topic is still relatively recent. Our understanding of the role of inflammation on depression still poses a lot of unanswered questions. Depression is a mental health problem that can be caused by multiple factors and is not completely understood by explaining this one mechanism. It is just this link of inflammation and its potential to promote symptoms of depression that we must understand if we are to treat depressive disorders more effectively and improve the future of healthcare, in particular, psychiatric outcomes. It

TABLE 3. Anti-inflammatory foods and how they help*

Anti-inflammatory Foods — Eat more	
Foods	**Why eat more**
Nuts and seeds: walnuts, chia seeds, hemp seeds, ground flaxseed or flax oil	Provide omega-3 fatty-acids, anti-inflammatory effects
Fatty fish: salmon, sardines, tuna, mackerel, trout, herring ***most fatty fish should be limited to 2-3 servings/week due to mercury contamination* ***generally, the higher up on food chain, the higher the contamination of mercury for particular fish; salmon and tuna are about in the middle of the food chain while shark or swordfish higher in the food chain, considered more contaminated*	
Avocados and legumes: beans, lentils, soybeans, and peas	Great sources of fiber, provide various amounts of essential fats, and provide antioxidants and other phytonutrients
Brightly colored vegetables and fruits (especially yellow, orange, red, and green): • carrots, bell peppers, tomatoes, broccoli, etc. Dark leafy greens/vegetables: • spinach, kale, collards, etc. Citrus fruits and berries: • Oranges, limes, lemon, etc. • Blueberries, blackberries, raspberries, strawberries, etc.	High in antioxidants, high in fiber; both can help promote anti-inflammatory effects
Various spices/herbs: • cayenne, clove, ginger, nutmeg, oregano, rosemary, turmeric	Provide various anti-inflammatory compounds or properties

*Adapted from *University of Wisconsin, Department of Family Medicine, Integrative Medicine Patient Handout* is the diet, in particular, and lifestyle factors, in general, that you have the ability to control. Over time, this can have profound effects on your health and improve the odds of brighter health in your future by "cooling the fires" in your body if it happens to be in a state of chronic inflammation.

PART II

GUT-BRAIN AXIS AND HOW TO MAINTAIN IT

He that takes medicine and neglects diet, wastes the time of his doctor.

ANCIENT CHINESE PROVERB

The doctor of the future will no longer treat the human frame with drugs, but rather will cure and prevent disease with nutrition.

THOMAS EDISON

CHAPTER 3

GUT HEALTH: GETTING TO KNOW YOUR FIRST AND SECOND BRAIN

GUT-BRAIN LINK

We've all heard something along the lines of "trust your gut", "butterflies in my stomach", or "... my gut feeling." In modern science, we're beginning to understand why it is common to express such intuitions or ardently voice a "gut feeling" about something. Besides the primary function of digesting food and absorbing nutrients, the gastrointestinal tract (gut) is supported by a complex network of neurons (nerve cells) that help the intestines function properly and "communicate" with the brain via chemical messengers (neurotransmitters). This network of nervous system tissue that facilitates communication between the gut and brain is often referred to as the "gut-brain axis" or "second brain", a term coined by Dr. Michael Gershon in 1996.[1]

As our understanding of gut health has rapidly advanced in the past couple of decades, we now know that other factors, such as maintaining gut barrier integrity and a robust, diverse gut microbiome, are critical for overall health and mental well-being. I will explore these factors and discuss how a healthy diet can help reduce your chances of harming these measures of gut health and, in turn, promote the health of your second brain and even protect or improve your mood. For those who already deal with serious gastrointestinal disorders or who have not yet determined the cause of ongoing digestive health problems, I'll discuss steps to tap into the natural healing processes of the body in a more holistic manner. This is different from simply treating the symptoms and masking the true cause of the problem.

The second brain pertains to the complex system of over 100 million neurons (the enteric nervous system) that surround and support the digestive tract. That's more nerve cells than are found in the spinal cord or the peripheral nervous system (other nerves that connect from the spinal cord to the rest of the body).[2] The enteric nervous system regulates the digestion and absorption of foods, biological waste elimination and, when not supported by a nutritious diet, can have a major impact on mental health and ability to lose or gain weight. This second brain, "hidden" within the wall of the intestinal tract, acts as a channel that sends and receives messages to the brain by way of the spinal cord and chemical messengers called neurotransmitters and hormones. These chemical messengers help to pass messages between neurons on their way to and from the brain.[3] However, the strength or clarity of this channel is dependent on a balanced, nutrient-dense diet. If you eat a "standard American diet", you are not likely to provide your body with the micronutrients required to adequately produce these neurotransmitters and allow this channel to have a clear signal and better communication with the brain.

Perhaps the biggest lesson to learn from the recent advance of gut health research is that the more we promote gut health or heal pre-existing gastrointestinal conditions, the more likely we are to see improvements with digestion, weight loss or maintenance, and overall mental well-being. If you have a digestive disorder that negatively affects your physical health and mental well-being, through a combination of diet, physical activity, stress management, and medications (as needed), you can achieve life-changing improvements. Making these changes and healing the gut is a complicated, yet powerful, process. For more details about gut-healing plans, some resources are mentioned at the end of the book.

Besides these important benefits to digestive health and overall physical health, I'll continue to explore the undeniable link between gut health and mental health. Let's not forget that physical health and mental health should not be separated because they are so critically linked. Later in this chapter I'll explore different lifestyle factors that impact your gut health, and in turn, your mental health. But first, take some time to learn a little about the normal function and health of the gastrointestinal tract.

DIGESTIVE/GUT HEALTH CRASH COURSE

Before making any lifestyle changes, it's important to be clear about *why*. Stop to pay a little respect to a normal functioning gastrointestinal tract and to the bugs (bacteria or microbes) that live on and inside every single one of us. From the moment you are brought into the world, leaving your mother's birth canal, you are exposed to billions of microscopic bacterial organisms. Some of the bacteria you're exposed to regularly are potentially harmful, some are beneficial and cover the surface area of the body, and others are more neutral or have no remarkable effects. With a healthy immune system, the body can usually fight off various sorts of potential infection from exposure to harmful bacteria one is normally exposed to. In fact, trillions of these microbes populate the inner lining of your intestines (among other areas of the body)! It is these friendly gut microbes that are proving to be a critical factor in improving overall health and moods.

Digestion

Food must be broken down into smaller fragmented pieces in order for nutrients to be released and absorbed later in the gastrointestinal tract. This process begins in the mouth with the process of chewing foods and stimulation of salivary enzymes that begin to break down strands of carbohydrates or starches. Then, digestion occurs in the stomach and the small intestine and is facilitated by digestive enzymes mostly from the pancreas, but also from the stomach and small intestine. Normal digestion is required for the body to extract nutrients from the food particles in the gastrointestinal tract. Without proper digestion, this will limit the body's ability to absorb key nutrients like calcium, magnesium, and iron. Digestive problems can impact physical health in many ways, including impairing the absorption of these nutrients.

Carbohydrates are broken down into glucose, which fuels all of the body's working cells and is the primary source of fuel for brain cells. Proteins are broken down into amino acids used to produce neurotransmitters and enzymes that speed up biochemical reactions. These digested amino acids have numerous other functions in the body and they are the building blocks for various forms of tissue structures. Dietary fats are broken down into smaller, free fatty acids (each molecule of fat is made up of fatty acids attached to a backbone molecule of glycerol) and provide an abundant source of energy (high in calories or "energy-dense").

Absorption

Once foods are broken down into more basic, elemental forms, they can be absorbed into the intestinal cells and then the bloodstream to then be taken into all of the working cells of the body. Although some absorption begins to occur in the stomach — alcohol and a few trace minerals like iodide and copper are absorbed in the stomach — the majority of absorption occurs throughout the intestines, with most nutrients being absorbed in the upper portion of the small intestine (referred to as the duodenum and the jejunum). Some gastrointestinal diseases, such as celiac disease, can damage the absorptive lining of the small intestine and impede absorption, which eventually can be a life-threatening disease if not managed by completely eliminating gluten from the diet (more on celiac and gluten in the next chapter).

Probiotics

Remember that live microorganisms or microbes naturally live on and inside the body. Particularly important are the community of gut microbes that inhabit the lining of the intestine, which is referred to as the gut microbiome (see definition below). In dietary terms, probiotics refer to the good bacteria that can be ingested through foods and supplements and then have beneficial effects on the human "host" — whether to form a sort of defense barrier in the intestines or to fortify the immune system in other ways. Probiotics not only help protect the immune system but they can also promote proper digestion of foods, prevent infection, diarrhea, and are even linked with preventing inflammation.[4] Probiotics have other important functions that we will explore later in Chapters 4 and 5. In this book, we'll also refer to probiotics as "good gut bugs" or "good bacteria."

Prebiotics

Prebiotics are a source of fuel for the good bacteria that populate the gut lining. Basically, prebiotics are various sources of dietary fibers that we can't digest but the good bacteria in the colon (large intestine) can digest and use to their benefit and in turn, your benefit! This is one of many reasons why a healthy diet should almost always (with a few exceptions, discussed in Chapter 4) include a variety of high-fiber foods, such as fruits, vegetables, whole grains, legumes, nuts, and seeds. More on prebiotics later in this chapter (*It's a Bug's Life)*.

Antibiotics

Since the discovery of penicillin in the late 1920s, various antibiotics have been life-saving for many different deadly diseases and are still readily used in medical practice. Besides the necessary and important role that antibiotics serve in medicine today, we must take note of the effect that these medicines also have on the healthy bacteria that inhabit the gastrointestinal tract. To simplify a complex matter, note that excessive usage of antibiotics may increase the likelihood of developing other health problems later in life, which are likely the result of reduced microbiological diversity and therefore decreased immune function in the gut. An interesting book that explains this problem in great detail is *Missing Microbes* by Dr. Martin Blaser.[5]

Microbiome (sometimes also referred to as microflora or microbiota)

Microbiome refers to the entirety of microorganisms (microbes) or genetic material (bacteria, fungi, protozoa, and bacteriophages) inside and on the body. In this chapter we will be focusing on the gut microbiome — particularly on bacteria and fungi that live inside the gut — as this is a key area that is implicated in a variety of different chronic illnesses and even in different mood disorders.[6] In particular, diversity of microorganisms is important to make sure we are adequately "fueling" the strains of bacteria that have health benefits. More on this in the next section.

MICROBIOME BALANCE: PROTECT YOUR INTERNAL ECOSYSTEM

Considering the whole body, there are approximately 30 trillion human cells. However, did you know that your body plays host to more than 100 trillion bacterial and fungal cells?[7] By some estimates, we have more than 10 times the amount of microbiological DNA within our bodies compared to our own genetic material. That's right, the majority of the DNA in the human body is from the microorganisms that reside on and inside each of us. In modern science, we now understand that our diet and lifestyle have a major impact on determining the diversity and healthfulness of one's "microbiome profile." It is the diversity of friendly gut bugs that we're learning is so important to not only promote a balanced and healthful gut microbiome but more broadly to help protect your "internal ecosystem" which makes up the majority of your immune system. That's right, approximately 70% of your entire immune system resides just below the layer of cells lining and protecting your intestinal cell wall.[8] So, if you don't take good care of your gut health through a varied diet, you are more likely to have a weak immune system (or perhaps an overstimulated immune system leading to other problems) and get sick more often with colds and infections.

Not all microbes that populate the gut are the same type or strain. It's estimated there are 10's of thousands of different strains of bacteria found in the genetic profile of humans.[9] Certain strains have beneficial effects in the body and for simplicity's sake, we will refer to them as healthy or good bacteria or "good gut bugs." Also, there are certain strains that may have negative effects on health when allowed to thrive, say from a high-stress lifestyle accompanied by a poor diet. The large intestine or colon alone has approximately 500 different bacterial species.[10] When you provide fuel for the various strains of friendly gut bugs by eating a variety of wholesome and fiber-rich plant-based foods, this promotes a diverse community of health-promoting microbes to populate the gut wall and protect your health. When the friendly gut bugs thrive, they serve important roles like promoting normal digestive health and manufacturing some vitamins, neurotransmitters, and anti-inflammatory chemicals. And perhaps most importantly for long-term health, these healthy microbes act as a "wall of defense" and serve as a barrier to the digestive tract to help assist the body with protecting a normal functioning immune system. In other words, a healthy diet is critical to allow particular beneficial microbes to thrive in certain areas of the intestinal tract while preventing other unfriendly bacterial strains or pathogens from taking up residence and flourishing in the gut. This is but one important factor to promote a balanced gut microbiome.

A balanced microbiome can help fight systemic inflammation and protect your gut-barrier (discussed in the next chapter). In turn, it can help with weight loss or weight maintenance, and can even have an impact on your mood, providing relief from symptoms of depression or anxiety. Part of these effects can be explained by the metabolic byproducts (end products of normal metabolism) of certain good gut bugs. Various foods with non-digestible carbohydrates (fiber) serve as fuel sources for these good bacteria. Although we can't digest the dietary fibers, they are fermented by the bacteria in the gut in order to produce short-chain fatty acids (SCFAs). These SCFAs communicate with the brain and may help fight inflammation. Even more notable, the SCFAs help nourish and turnover the cells of the intestinal lining (called enterocytes), and protect the barrier of the intestines.[11] When we cool the fires of chronic inflammation and facilitate normal digestive health through a diverse and balanced gut microbiome, over time this is likely to result in improvements in body weight and mood.

On the other hand, if you eat a "standard American diet" (SAD), you may be starving the good bacteria while promoting the growth of certain bacteria or even fungal strains with undesirable effects. If left uncorrected, this can eventually lead to other serious digestive or gut-health problems (discussed in the next chapter). Low diversity and amount of good bacteria, along with proliferation or overgrowth of bad bacteria, contribute to an unbalanced microbiome. This is also referred to as dysbiosis and may negatively impact many different aspects of health. Beyond digestive problems, gut dysbiosis is linked with attention deficit hyperactivity disorder (ADHD), allergies, autism, autoimmune disorders, Alzheimer's disease, and mood disorders, such as schizophrenia, bipolar disorder, and major depressive disorder.[12,13] The autoimmune disorders linked with dysbiosis include celiac disease, type 1 diabetes, multiple sclerosis, and rheumatoid arthritis.[14] Although research is still too early and uncertain to make any determinations about cause and effect, some researchers suspect that a chronically inflamed gut, along with gut dysbiosis, may even help explain the onset of some of these diseases.

Dysbiosis is more likely to occur in people who don't have a healthy lifestyle. Particularly, those who eat little-to-no plant-based whole foods, don't manage stress well, have poor sleep quality, and don't regularly participate in any sort of physical activity. Unfortunately, these all too often go hand-in-hand with each other. Too much of these unfriendly bacteria in your gut ecosystem is strongly linked with increased gas, bloating, painful stools, chronic constipation, and diarrhea. For many people, these common complaints are often diagnosed as irritable bowel syndrome (IBS).

Although the exact cause of IBS is not well known, there is a growing body of evidence that suggests it is dysbiosis — an unbalanced gut microbiome — that is the major contributor to IBS. As mentioned previously, we also know that dysbiosis is a contributing factor to the dysfunction of the immune system and inflammation of the nervous system tissue. In turn, these factors increase the chances of developing diseases of the brain.[15] Knowing how these gut bugs contribute to gut-health, brain-health and overall-health and quality of life, it's no wonder that an unbalanced gut microbiome can contribute to, not necessarily cause, a poor mood or depression.

IT'S A BUG'S LIFE

The microflora or microbiome in your gut is sometimes compared to a garden that needs to be maintained, similar to how you might care for a garden at home. If you want to avoid too many weeds growing, prevent all the pretty plants and produce from dying, and keep the grass green, then you need to spend some time and care for your garden. Now, imagine what happens when you fail to care for that garden: over time the weeds and pests take over the yard and the desirable flowers and produce die off. This lack of caring for the garden outside is similar to the effects of eating a standard American diet paired with a high-stress lifestyle on your gut microbiome. We need to take better care of the good gut bugs.

Some of the nutrients that the good bacteria produce may also help to improve energy or mood. B-vitamins are required to convert food into energy and to produce neurotransmitters that regulate mood and need to be consumed throughout the diet. Unlike bacteria, yeasts, or even plants, humans cannot make their own B vitamins. For good health and energy, we need a steady supply of these in our diet, along with what's contributed to the body from the good gut bugs. When you eat a balanced and varied diet, some of the fibers in foods (prebiotics) fuel these healthy bacteria, and, in turn, these gut bugs help produce nutrients such as vitamin K, short-chain fatty acids (SCFAs, discussed above), and B-vitamins folate, B-12, and biotin among others.[16,17] These B-vitamins also play important protective roles in health due to helping stimulate and support the normal function of the immune system and nervous system. However, not all bacterial strains can produce these vitamins and so it's important to eat a balanced and varied diet, including a variety of fibrous plant-based whole foods, to encourage more diverse strains of healthy bacteria to take up residence in the gut.

Not only are vitamins and anti-inflammatory properties produced by gut microbes, but some of the important neurotransmitters that regulate mood are also produced by these good gut bugs. Different strains of good bacteria in the gut produce serotonin, dopamine, gamma-amino butyrate (GABA), and norepinephrine.[18] Neurotransmitters are like chemical messengers between nerve cells. Serotonin, an important neurotransmitter that regulates mood — and even plays a role in digestive processes, sleep cycle, and immune responses — is mostly produced within the intestines and its normal production is somewhat dependent on a nutritious diet. By some estimates, 90% or more of serotonin is produced in the gut. Besides what's produced by the good bacteria, much of the serotonin is produced by specialized cells in the gut, such as "enterochromaffin cells" and "mucosal mast cells."[19] Some of the friendly microbes, such as lactic acid bacteria, help to produce gamma-aminobutyric acid (GABA), an important calming neurotransmitter that signals to inhibit or slow the central nervous system, thereby inducing a calming, antianxiety effect.[20] Acetylcholine, another neurotransmitter important for memory, attention, and motivation, is also produced by this species of bacteria.[21]

We're only beginning to understand how essential a nutrient-dense, balanced diet is to promoting gut health and preventing chronic diseases. When making healthy diet changes, we must keep in mind that *it's a bug's life*! That is, the health and diversity of the good gut bugs that inhabit the gastrointestinal tract are directly related to your health. Some would argue they rule our health. In turn, a diverse and balanced gut microbiome promotes the health of the brain, our moods, and overall mental wellbeing. When flourishing, the good bacteria help prevent overcrowding and pathogens and the bad bacteria from flourishing and wreaking havoc on your health. When left uncorrected, a disrupted gut microbiome accompanied by an unhealthy lifestyle, can eventually lead to a breakdown of the protective lining of the gut. For those who deal with complex gut health problems, Chapter 4 dives deeper into some of the most common and frustrating among them.

CHAPTER 4

CARE FOR YOUR SECOND BRAIN: A DEEPER LOOK

N ow that you have a better appreciation for the relationship between your brain and your gut (the second brain), let's discuss some of the factors that contribute to poor gut health and the most important things you must do to take good care of your gut health. Let's also review some of the most common gastrointestinal disorders that commonly present barriers or obstacles to many people when trying to eat a healthy diet and make lifestyle changes. When you address these barriers first, it is only then that you can achieve lasting, life-changing results. This chapter is particularly relevant for those who currently have a gastrointestinal disorder and have had multiple unsuccessful attempts at dietary changes in the past. Lastly, this chapter will outline what integrative and functional medicine (IFM) practitioners refer to as a "gut healing protocol."

Besides doctors, IFM practitioners can also include many different types of medical professionals such as physician's assistants, physical therapists, occupational therapists, chiropractors, registered dietitians, or other types of clinicians who have completed specialized education and requirements. For example, The Institute for Functional Medicine is one of the leading organizations that educates and certifies medical practitioners in this specialized form of practicing medicine and lifestyle changes. This chapter will guide you in the right direction in case you need to address a GI disorder and seek out an IFM practitioner before following general healthful dietary recommendations.

GUT-BARRIER INTEGRITY

Besides the critical role of digesting and absorbing foods, the intestines play a protective role in preventing pathogens, undigested food particles, or other non-food particles from getting into the bloodstream. The "gut barrier" is composed of tight junctions between intestinal cells called enterocytes. These tight junctions that basically lock cells to one another with their neighboring cells, help form a barrier and normally prevent most non-food substances, toxins, or undigested food materials from passing into the bloodstream from inside the intestinal tract and triggering an immune system reaction. When the structure of this cellular barrier is damaged by chronic inflammation and disrupted gut microbiome, this signals the immune system to be on alert and attack whatever foreign invaders might enter the bloodstream and so an immune response follows.

When the integrity of this gut barrier is breached or damaged, this is referred to as increased intestinal permeability (IP). Some people (not usually medical practitioners) refer to this phenomenon as "leaky gut syndrome" because of the potential for harmful substances to "leak" into the body and trigger a defense response. Over time, this may increase the chances of developing allergies and autoimmune diseases. This increased IP is also directly related to chronic inflammation of the gut, which as we have already identified may be a compelling cause or contributing factor of major depression.[1] When the gut barrier is chronically inflamed and there's a lack of healthy gut bugs available, this can impede the body's ability to absorb nutrients. Nutrient malabsorption can complicate other health problems and often this must be addressed in order to correct underlying medical conditions.

A variety of lifestyle and dietary factors and even certain medications may increase the likelihood of your gut barrier becoming compromised.

Some evidence suggests that gluten (a type of protein found in certain grains like wheat) may promote increased IP.[2,3] This may explain why it's becoming more common to have a sensitivity (intolerance) to gluten and wheat products while not having celiac disease, a more specific diagnosis that is better understood and treated by a strict gluten elimination diet. Other factors that may contribute to increased intestinal permeability are: a low intake of dietary fiber (most Americans eat about half of the recommended daily amount!); excessive intake of alcohol; stress; and an overall poor diet and unhealthy lifestyle which can promote the proliferation of bad bacteria and inflammation of the gut.

Certain types of medications, especially when overused, can negatively impact the microbiome and contribute to increased intestinal permeability. Some of these common medications include antibiotics, proton-pump inhibitors ("PPIs"; a common class of medications for acid reflux, peptic ulcer, abdominal discomfort, and indigestion), birth control medications[4], and NSAIDs (non-steroidal anti-inflammatory drugs, including various over-the-counter pain medication).[5,6] Besides the life-saving potential of antibiotics to "kill off" the bad bacterial strains that cause different illnesses, they also kill off the good bacteria and may eventually contribute to compromised gut-barrier integrity. Likewise, medications for indigestion or acid reflux may offer people much-needed relief from troubling symptoms. However, treating these conditions with such medications does not always effectively treat the underlying condition, rather it treats the symptoms of the disease, while long-term usage may contribute to other health problems. This is not at all to suggest that these medications should not be used. These medications serve an important purpose for many people. If, for example, you've taken many different courses of antibiotics in the past or used NSAIDS or PPIs for extended periods of time and you experience serious gut health issues, then this is a clue that you may have a low diversity of good gut bacteria and too much bad bacteria overgrowing, impacting the integrity of the gut barrier.

On the other hand, metformin — one of the most commonly prescribed drugs for new-onset diabetes —helps control blood sugar and is believed to have a beneficial impact on the gut microbiome for some. How this medication works on the microbiome is not well understood. However, recent evidence suggests that a modification of the number of different strains of bacteria in the gut may help explain why this drug is so helpful for regulating blood sugar.[7] This is further evidence that *It's a bug's life.* In other words, if you don't pay enough respect to the health of your resident gut bugs, you're not respecting your gut-barrier integrity and, consequently, your overall physical and mental health.

GOT GUT HEALTH ISSUES? KNOW THE PROBLEM BEFORE TAKING ACTION!

A quote from Joshua Fields Milburn, "The Minimalists" podcast, illustrates the importance of this chapter: "[We need to] put the fire out first before we rebuild the house." This speaks to the importance of addressing any gut inflammation, dysbiosis, or other complications that may need to be treated prior to achieving lifelong success from diet changes. Common medical conditions to address prior to making general healthful dietary changes are:

- Irritable bowel syndrome (IBS)
- Inflammatory bowel disease (IBD) - Crohn's disease, ulcerative colitis
- Other inflammatory conditions such as gastritis or diverticulitis
- Gastroparesis or other serious gastrointestinal disorders, such as small bowel obstructions or other rare conditions that must be addressed by a specialized doctor or gastroenterologist
- Food allergies or intolerances

If you suffer from distressing gastrointestinal (GI) symptoms on a regular or daily basis, then it's very important to properly determine the root cause of GI disorder before making any major lifestyle changes. This might be the only way to find something more than temporary relief — what is commonly offered as a treatment for many with undiagnosed, or even misdiagnosed, gut health disorders. This is a common frustration I hear expressed from too many patients who have consulted me in healthcare clinics. That is, it's common to be treated for certain GI disorders and get help with temporary relief of symptoms; however, some medications don't address the underlying cause. So these conditions tend to either resurface later or sometimes even contribute to other more concerning health problems down the line.

Unfortunately, many doctors in conventional Western medicine or standard American healthcare may not be aware of how to treat the underlying causes of many of these conditions or are simply unaware of the more nuanced understanding of the likely causes and the treatment protocols that do exist. Although, healing the gut is outside the scope of this book, the good news is that there are many integrative and functional medicine (IFM) practitioners and other qualified practitioners, such as experienced registered dietitians (RDN or RD credentials) and nutritionists with specialized training in integrative and functional medicine, who can help you heal your gut. In simple terms, integrative and functional medicine entails a more holistic model of healthcare that aims to get to the root cause of different diseases. Unlike traditional medicine in the U.S., IFM is a clinical approach adopted by certain doctors and other medical practitioners, which includes working closely with the patient, establishing a detailed account of the patient's history and lifestyle to provide individualized care, and also using the expertise of a variety of different (integrated) healthcare specialties.

IBS vs. IBD

Irritable bowel syndrome (IBS) is a common medical condition that affects the quality of life of far too many people. Estimates suggest about 15% of Americans are impacted by IBS. Whether it is marked by chronic constipation, chronic diarrhea, or both, IBS can affect people in different ways. This medical condition is characterized by a change in the consistency and/or frequency of bowel movements accompanied by abdominal pain or discomfort. Common complaints include bloating, gas/indigestion, and irregular or painful bowel movements. Although the exact cause is not well understood, it's believed that some of the biggest contributing factors to IBS are stress, disrupted gut motility (muscle contractions in the gut that keep things moving along), and diet which has a subsequent effect on the balance and diversity of bacteria in the gut.[8] Interestingly, each of these factors relates to the almighty gut bugs!

Inflammatory bowel disease (IBD) refers to a variety of different chronic diseases that are characterized by chronic inflammation of different sections of the gut. Most commonly, this includes Crohn's disease and ulcerative colitis, which affect the small intestine (primarily) and the colon, respectively. Not everybody with these conditions is affected the same way; typical symptoms include abdominal pain or cramping, diarrhea, fever, unintentional weight loss, and sometimes rectal bleeding which may indicate other potentially more concerning gastrointestinal problems.[9] The duration of time that one endures pain and discomfort can vary widely from person to person. Some people only occasionally have painful "flare-ups" from time to time, while others may experience painful and unpleasant symptoms more regularly. Because some of the symptoms of IBD are similar to those one might experience with irritable bowel syndrome (IBS), there's a chance that a physician may misdiagnose symptoms as a case of IBS, a less well-understood and less specific diagnosis, when the person might actually have IBD, a more troubling but better understood diagnosis with a clearer treatment plan. This is one example of how an integrative & functional medicine doctor would likely have greater insight than most conventionally trained physicians.

It's important to distinguish between gut health conditions because there are different strategies to address each of these and they're briefly discussed in the last section of this chapter. Furthermore, if left untreated IBD may eventually lead to other potentially life-threatening conditions. Depending on the particular diagnosis and situation, doctors may recommend surgery to remove sections of the intestines.

Other Inflammatory and Miscellaneous Gut Health Disorders

Besides the chronic inflammatory bowel diseases (IBD) discussed above, there are other inflammatory conditions and gut health disorders that can result in similar symptoms but may tend to come and go from time to time. For example, approximately 50% of people develop pouch-like "diverticula" in the large intestine (colon) after age 50. Although diverticula don't always cause problems, these abnormally-formed pouches in the colon can become inflamed and result in painful and distressing symptoms, some of which are similar to what's experienced in those with IBD. When the diverticula become inflamed, the condition is considered diverticulitis and requires a different treatment compared to when the pouches are not inflamed. Typically, diverticulitis is treated with antibiotics and a low fiber diet to help reduce painful symptoms. However, this treatment doesn't necessarily address the underlying cause of the inflammatory condition. By this point, you can imagine that multiple treatment rounds of antibiotics along with a low fiber diet is not going to do much good over time for promoting a balanced microbiome, and consequently, not much good for long-term gut health.

Other common gastrointestinal diseases that may require special care from your doctor include gastritis (inflammation of the stomach lining), peptic ulcers, or bacterial disease in the stomach (referred to as an H. pylori infection). Helicobacter pylori (H. pylori) is a type of bacteria that is linked to stomach cancer and peptic ulcer disease and is believed to be the main cause of chronic gastritis.[10] Interestingly, however, there's evidence that humans have carried this strain of bacteria for at least 100,000 years and that having this bacteria in the stomach does not always result in gastritis, peptic ulcers, or even stomach cancer. Among the most respected researchers on the subject of H. pylori, Dr. Martin Blaser suggests that to rid the body of H. pylori, through the treatment of antibiotics and other medications, may result in other long-term health problems for some people. In *Missing Microbes*, Dr. Blaser states that "H. pylori play a role in the production of acid and hormones and the state of immunity."[11] Estimates suggest that at least 50% of Americans have this type of bacteria in their stomach, yet many of these people have no health problems related to it. In fact, only about 15–20% of people who have H. pylori will develop an ulcer.[12] This might be explained by the fact that normal production of stomach acid keeps this level of H. pylori in check and thus prevents it from causing damage to the stomach lining and a subsequent inflammatory response that could contribute to gastritis, among other health problems. Dr. Blaser states, "H. pylori strains possess a protein that in sufficient quantity pokes holes in the epithelial cells that line the stomach wall."[13] Perhaps the take-home message here is that there are some potential health benefits to humans from hosting H. pylori bacteria in the stomach. More importantly, however, this bacteria can also be harmful when it is provided with the right conditions to grow too much or cause an infection.

When the normal production of stomach acid is disrupted, this can lead to other more serious gut health conditions over time. This highlights another shortcoming in our understanding of how to properly treat the underlying causes of various gut health problems. Currently, the primary mode of treating H. pylori infection is by "triple therapy", which includes two different antibiotics and a proton-pump inhibitor (PPI). Although triple therapy may provide a much-needed relief from symptoms of H. pylori infection, the long-term concerns may not be worth the risk. Some patients might prefer to explore more complementary and integrated treatment options.

Over the long-term, frequent use of antibiotics, along with the proton-pump inhibitors that suppress the natural production of stomach acid, can increase the chances of developing indigestion and malabsorption of nutrients. PPIs are usually only indicated for use up to 4–8 weeks, while they're often used for longer periods of time. For example, long-term use of PPIs is associated with impaired absorption of magnesium and vitamin B-12 and may contribute to deficient levels of these critically important nutrients. When used for extended periods of time or with multiple courses, PPIs and antibiotics are also linked with a higher chance of developing gut dysbiosis and troubling conditions such as small intestinal bacterial overgrowth (SIBO) or small intestinal fungal overgrowth (SIFO).[14]

SIBO and SIFO

Did you know that there are different amounts and types of bacteria and fungi strains, or different communities of microorganisms in different sections of your gastrointestinal tract? For the most part, the good gut bugs (and bad bacteria) live and function in the large intestine and much less so in the small intestine area. However, sometimes bacteria grow excessively in places where their presence is supposed to be limited, such as the small intestine. Remember, the main job of the small intestine is to absorb nutrients, so the gut bugs should not be nearly as densely-populated here as compared to the large intestine. Among other contributing factors, such as certain medications, this bacterial overgrowth in undesirable areas can occur from a lack of sufficient stimulation or movement of the gastrointestinal tract. The normal sequence of contractions and movement of the intestinal tract is called motility, and is very important for the normal function of a healthy digestive tract.

The medical condition referred to as SIBO (small intestinal bacterial overgrowth) results from too much bacteria overpopulating the small intestine. This off-balance can interfere with the normal function of the small intestine. Common symptoms include abdominal pain, bloating, nausea, fatigue, constipation, and diarrhea. In more severe cases, the absorptive capacity of the small intestine may be impacted and this can lead to anemia or other nutrient deficiencies. SIBO is usually treated with antibiotics and many people find short-lived relief with symptoms. However, it's not uncommon for SIBO to come back and pose the same problems as before if the root problems are not addressed. This may include addressing a poor diet, poor digestive tract movement, or other less common medical complications.[15]

Similar to SIBO, potentially dangerous overgrowths of fungal strains can also occur and pose similar health concerns. This is referred to as small intestinal fungal overgrowth (SIFO). However, SIFO is not as well researched as SIBO and so it's just not quite as well recognized or understood. One study showed that out of 150 patients that visited the same gastrointestinal (GI) doctor over a 15-year period, 94 of them (about 63%) tested positive for either SIBO or SIFO. Out of the 94 people with intestinal overgrowth, about 60% tested the positive for either SIFO or both of these conditions.[16]

Are you noticing a common theme here? As with the gut health conditions discussed earlier, the important note here speaks to the role of a diverse and balanced gut microbiome in order to help your body's biological systems stay in check. We need this diverse community of bacteria, in the right places, to stay in a state of internal balance or homeostasis.

Indigestion and GERD

Indigestion (dyspepsia) refers to a variety of symptoms that often cluster together, including abdominal discomfort, bloating, nausea, or even feeling full too quickly after eating. This is a signal that the body and GI tract are not doing a very good job of digesting foods properly. Acid reflux — marked by heartburn or a burning sensation in the throat — is common and experienced by most people from time to time. However, some people experience this problem more frequently and this may indicate something more concerning, such as a chronic problem like gastroesophageal reflux disease (GERD).

Although dietary factors play a big part in normal healthy digestion, let's not forget about stress! We discussed earlier how harmful stress can be to one's health in general. But in particular, stress can be harmful to digestive health. Stress diminishes digestive function by reducing the secretion of digestive enzymes, in essence turning off the digestion light switch. Furthermore, impaired digestion can affect the production of the neurotransmitters that regulate your mood, sleep quality, and food cravings or appetite. High stress can also impact the gastrointestinal tract by inducing esophageal spasms (hiccups), increased stomach acid and heartburn, nausea, constipation, or diarrhea.[17]

For those who live chronically stressed lives, the body's sympathetic nervous system may be overstimulated, while the parasympathetic nervous system is deactivated. Basically, this means that the "fight or flight" warning system of the body is working overtime, preventing the body from entering "rest and restore" mode, and subsequently impacting normal digestive processes. To avoid confusion, let's keep the discussion limited to the basics of these opposing physiological processes. In simple terms, the parasympathetic nervous system is also known as the "rest and digest" or "rest and restore" system. When the opposite, "fight or flight" system is on overdrive, this prevents the "rest and digest" system from working. If you have poor digestion, high stress, and don't practice self-care measures or manage the daily stressors that you encounter, then it's no wonder that the normal digestive processes light switch is shut off or at least dimmed. Without adequate rest, the production of stomach acid and digestive enzymes may be affected which then affects the digestion and absorption of foods and nutrients. In normal health, the body maintains a dynamic balance of these two systems. Therefore, stress management is one more tool for improving treatments for a variety of different gastrointestinal issues that may either be caused by, or at least exacerbated by, stress. Other factors to consider that may limit one's ability to relax and impair digestion are excessive smoking, caffeine, and alcohol consumption.

Food Allergies, Intolerances, and Autoimmune Disorders

As you can tell, an unhealthy or unbalanced gut microbiome is related to a wide variety of health conditions, even beyond the discussion in this book. If we take a closer look at the likely root causes of GI disorders discussed above, the body's natural defense mechanisms have become faulty in most cases, or turned on us, causing harm rather than preventing it. Normal digestive health is required to keep these natural defense mechanisms in check, but more generally, to regulate a normal immune system. Can you believe that even food allergies and various autoimmune disorders are related to the diet and a disrupted gut microbiome?

It's common to confuse the two or even think that food allergies and intolerances are one and the same. However, they are unique biological responses occurring in the body and you should note the difference. A food *allergy* is marked by the natural response of the immune system trying to attack the "foreign invader" protein molecule (food particle) that the body has developed an allergic response to. This can either be a protein that the body doesn't recognize as normal but still triggers an immune response to, or it can be a known allergy that your body has already been exposed to and has developed a more orchestrated and powerful immune response to. The reactions to a food allergy range in severity and usually occur abruptly, within a few minutes or up to a couple of hours after exposure to the food allergen. Symptoms can include (but are not limited to) tingling or itching of the mouth, swelling of the lips, tongue, throat, or other areas, and even abdominal pain, diarrhea, nausea, and vomiting.[18]

Some of the most common foods that people are allergic to include milk, eggs, fish, shellfish, peanuts, tree nuts, wheat, and soy. These are often referred to as "the Big-8" because they're recognized as the most common food allergens and are responsible for approximately 90% of all food allergies in the U.S.[19]

Food *intolerances* are different from allergies because the body's immune system is not responding to the problematic food as it does to a food allergen. Likely occurring more often than food allergies, food intolerances are characterized by an inability to adequately digest or absorb certain foods. An intolerance to a food is a sign of a poor digestive response to that type of food. One of the more common and well-known food intolerances is lactose intolerance. Also common, yet less understood, is fructose intolerance.

Fructose is a natural sugar found in fruits and some vegetables. It is isolated from corn, and produced in mass quantities to make high-fructose corn syrup, an ingredient found in processed foods. Fructose intolerance is a problem that affects many people, yet may be overlooked or even misdiagnosed. People with lactose or fructose intolerance don't tolerate foods with these types of sugars because they either lack the particular enzyme(s) required to digest these sugars, or in some cases, may have an unbalanced gut microbiome.

Another common food intolerance is gluten intolerance. Note that gluten intolerance is not the same thing as celiac disease, where a person is not able to digest the type of protein called gluten found in wheat and other grains. Unlike celiac disease in which gluten triggers an immune system response, the root cause of gluten intolerance is not well understood.

Lactose or gluten intolerance is relatively simple to address by targeting and avoiding products containing gluten and avoiding most dairy products. However, fructose intolerance or malabsorption can be more challenging or confusing to address due to how many foods naturally contain fructose. Not to mention all the processed foods with lots of fructose added in the form of high fructose corn syrup. Between the years 1970 and 1990, Americans increased their consumption of high fructose corn syrup (HFCS) a staggering 1000%.[20] Also noteworthy is that both fructose malabsorption and lactose intolerance are linked with irritable bowel syndrome (IBS). Although we can't say definitively what the cause of IBS is, for some people, it's possible that these (or other) food intolerances might be a root cause, and by eliminating certain foods and resolving food intolerances, the common symptoms of bloating, abdominal discomfort, and diarrhea will likely go away.

Similar to small intestinal bacterial overgrowth (SIBO), fructose maldigestion and lactose intolerance can be diagnosed with breath testing from your doctor. This is a simple, non-invasive way to determine the degree to which you digest a particular type of carbohydrate-containing food after ingesting it. Specifically, this testing method measures the amount of gases in your breath produced after eating the problematic food. Gases, such as hydrogen and methane, that form from the undigested food passing into the large intestine promote symptoms such as abdominal discomfort, bloating, or diarrhea.[21] Besides the breath testing method done by doctors, you can also try a food elimination diet trial to determine which foods are part of a digestive problem. More on elimination diet trials in the final section of this chapter.

You may be thinking it's a long shot to make the connection between diet, food allergies and intolerances, and autoimmune disorders. However tenuous this link may be, it's important to note that both food allergies and autoimmune disorders are often a consequence of a dysfunctional immune system and, as you know by now, most of your immune system (about 70% or more of total immune-related tissue) resides within your gut.[22] This illustrates the importance of maintaining normal digestive gut health in order to maintain normal immune health. One of the important lessons of this book is that normal digestive and immunological function may reduce the chances of developing chronic and problematic dysfunction of the immune system such as autoimmune disorders.

What are autoimmune disorders? The term autoimmunity refers to the body's immune response against its own cells or tissues, rather than just attacking the usual foreign invaders in the bloodstream like a normally functioning immune system. To put it simply, an autoimmune disorder is when the body's own defense mechanism turns against itself. This is almost like groups of soldiers putting on their enemies' uniforms while at war and attacking their fellow soldiers. Although symptoms vary among different conditions, many autoimmune disorders share common symptoms, including fatigue, joint pain, and swelling, swollen glands, recurring fever, skin problems, abdominal pain, and digestive complications.[23] Some common autoimmune disorders are related to increased intestinal permeability or "leaky gut", including type 1 diabetes, multiple sclerosis, rheumatoid arthritis, and celiac disease.[24]

Though we already discussed the importance of maintaining gut-barrier integrity, it's mentioned again here because there are other types of immune system cells stored within and underneath the intestinal cells which form the main part of the gut-barrier. This layer of immune cells is beneath the protective outer layer of mucus and bacteria. When the protective outer layer of mucus and bacteria is disrupted and the tight junctions between the intestinal cells are weakened, this signals the immune system cells to begin producing different chemicals in preparation for the "attack" of the foreign invader that penetrated the protective outer layers.[25]

Although we cannot say for sure what the exact cause of an autoimmune disease like celiac disease is, there is evidence that in genetically susceptible people, dietary gluten causes an "upregulation" (increased biological production) of zonulin (a type of protein that is the only known molecule in the body that controls the tight junctions between the intestinal cells). In other words, in some people, gluten from grains like wheat may increase the likelihood of compromising the gut barrier. Despite the lack of clear understanding of the root causes of autoimmune diseases, the evidence is becoming clearer and suggesting that if we don't do a better job at protecting the microbiome balance and gut-barrier integrity, we are likely creating the perfect storm for chronic digestive problems and an overstimulated immune system.

Left unaddressed, eventually, this perfect storm may open the door up to more serious and complex health problems such as autoimmune diseases and a variety of mental health problems.

The point in this chapter is not to learn details about each of the conditions discussed, rather to highlight the importance of identifying the root cause of the particular gastrointestinal condition you may be experiencing. If you believe you're dealing with one or perhaps several of the conditions discussed above, there is not a one-size-fits-all approach and so it's important to work closely with your team of healthcare professionals to find answers about the root causes of your gastrointestinal problems. Once you know the root cause of your gut health problems, only then can you strategize the best approach towards healing your gut and finding lifelong solutions. These lifelong solutions might not only give you answers to your digestive problems, but you might also find that when your digestive problems clear up, you also notice improvements in overall quality of life and mental well-being.

GUT HEALING

The human body has an amazing ability to heal itself. However, when not given the right building blocks, fuel, and conditions to function optimally, it cannot use that ability well. We have previously suggested the importance of lifestyle factors in helping to promote overall health (see Afterword for self-care discussion). These factors play a critical role in helping the body maintain its normal healing capacity. Granted, the specific concept of "gut-healing" is somewhat controversial, theoretical, and not yet well-accepted by conventional medicine. But this does not negate the potential healing power that integrative and functional medicine practitioners are likely to understand and be able to offer as part of their medical practices.

You may have to seek out an integrative and functional medicine practitioner because many conventionally trained doctors do not have the advanced understanding of these gastrointestinal diseases needed to identify likely causes and contributing factors. Perhaps even more frustrating for some people, your gut health problems might get misdiagnosed or overlooked while a traditional physician focuses on other medical concerns.

After some careful consideration and a discussion with your doctor about your gut health issues, you may realize you might have a common case of gut dysbiosis and maybe even some increased intestinal permeability. Now what is there to do about it? While modifying your diet to promote good bacteria and limit bad bacteria may sound simple in theory, achieving it may not be so easy. More importantly, the solution is not simple, and there are things besides diet your medical provider might consider. Certain gut health conditions require modified protocols. It's important to get help from your doctor as you may need other tests or procedures.

The best advice for one person is not always best for everybody! Maybe you've tried many different diets or even modified your diet, and you know you just can't tolerate certain healthy foods, not to mention the disappointing lack of success. There may be a good reason you don't tolerate certain foods and haven't made progress with past diets. Maybe you need to take the time to learn which foods you can't tolerate, honor your body, and not eat those foods. Unfortunately, the basic advice to eat fruits, vegetables, and whole grains is not the right advice for people with certain conditions. In other words, if you suffer from certain digestive problems, the health of your "garden of gut microbes" might be a major barrier to making dietary changes you can stick with for life. Some medical conditions that might benefit from a tailored gut healing protocol include:

- Small intestinal bacterial overgrowth (SIBO)
- Small intestinal fungal overgrowth (SIFO)
- Inflammatory bowel diseases (IBDs), including Crohn's disease and ulcerative colitis
- Other inflammatory conditions such as gastritis or diverticulitis

Sometimes the appropriate diet recommendations for people with certain conditions are contrary to what's recommended to the general public. For example, people with inflammatory bowel disease (IBD) are recommended to follow a low-fiber diet to help reduce painful symptoms attributed to ingesting too many high-fiber foods. Also, those with irritable bowel syndrome (IBS) are commonly told to follow more specific recommendations about which high-fiber foods to eat and which to avoid or limit. One example of a diet that specifies which carbohydrate-containing foods can and cannot be included is the "low-FODMAP" diet. "FODMAPs" is short for Fermentable, Oligosaccharides, Disaccharides, Monosaccharides, and Polyols. In simpler terms, these are carbohydrates that the small intestine may absorb poorly.[26] Both the low-fiber and low FODMAP diets differ greatly from what's more commonly recommended and considered a healthful diet.

For those making significant dietary changes who also have certain gut health problems such as irritable bowel syndrome (IBS) or inflammatory bowel diseases (IBD), there are special tests and steps that may need to be completed prior to embarking on diet changes that are discussed in Part III of this book. In other words, there may be important medical business to take care of prior to finding lasting success with a general healthful diet. Don't be scared. Be patient as you take time to appreciate your daily choices and the power of lifestyle changes, and find your path to life-changing results.

What Does Not Work: A Note on Misinformation

Nutrition information in general can be confusing and oftentimes misleading. It's no wonder there's plenty of short-sighted information or misinformation all around about how to improve gut health conditions. If you look to the internet for answers about healing the root causes of your digestive problems, you might get lost in a jungle of information. There are endless amounts of misleading and unproven claims out there with suggestions to take this product or that product for relief. From the paleo diet to keto diet to carnivore diet, there are endless answers about what might help digestive health, yet some hold more promise than others and can be used more strategically. Whether it's apple cider vinegar, coconut oil, kombucha, bone broths, or probiotics, these are just a few products with often touted, yet minimally supported, health claims. I'm not saying these diets or products are not good for you, nor am I saying there are no potential health benefits from such foods or products. I am saying that these are not long-term solutions to complex gut health problems. They are certainly not a one-size-fits-all answer to different complex gut health conditions, despite some of these providing a benefit for some people. When somebody takes these products or follows a restrictive diet and doesn't otherwise modify their diet and lifestyle or take the necessary first steps with their medical providers, then the anticipated benefits of taking individual food products are likely never to be realized. The point here is that if you don't get to the root cause of what the digestive problem is, then it's hard to treat the underlying cause and ever find any lifelong relief.

What Does Work: Elimination Diet Trials

What does work and what can help you find answers and lasting solutions, is strictly following an elimination diet trial, maintaining a food diary and symptom log, and working closely with an experienced doctor that is specially trained in integrative and functional medicine. A doctor that will listen to your gastrointestinal complaints and take a strategic approach towards determining the root cause of whatever is ailing you and your digestive health can work for you. At the least, it can help you begin to find answers to health problems you haven't found before. And for those that have more complex digestive issues, you may need some additional tests or procedures to determine other necessary steps in your gut-healing journey.

One simple, cheap, and non-invasive way to determine if you have an intolerance to a food is to do a food elimination diet for a trial period of about four to six weeks. Those following an elimination diet should strictly avoid common (suspected or identified) trigger foods for a specific amount of time (such as a 21-day period) and then re-introduce them one-by-one while maintaining a detailed journal of dietary intake, noting thoughts and feelings or any symptoms experienced after eating those foods. This process of journaling will help you identify and track any patterns of symptoms. Sometimes the 21-days might not be long enough to notice considerable relief in symptoms. If no relief is noticed after such an elimination trial, then you might find some relief extending it up to four to six weeks. However, if no considerable relief is noticed after that long, it's probably a good indication there may be something else more complex going on that needs a closer look by a GI specialist (gastroenterologist) and/or integrative and functional medicine practitioner. There may be a need to treat bacterial or fungal overgrowth or inflammatory conditions. Further, there may be a need to repair the gut lining, possibly harmed by an unhealthy lifestyle.

Determining your best approach towards healing your gut is outside the scope of this book, though it's important for you to realize that

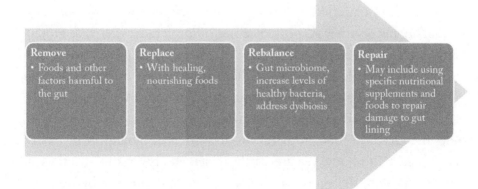

FIGURE 2. The Four R's of Gut Healing

there are answers out there for your complex gut health problems. You can find relief from your distressing symptoms. Although they might not be as easy-to-follow or easy-to-find answers as you would like them to be, lasting relief is worth the cost or effort and requires some patience.

Let's briefly explore the basic steps of a gut-healing protocol. One example is commonly referred to as the "Four R's of Gut Healing."

Phase 1 - Remove

This is about removing any dietary or other factors that could be major contributors to your gut health woes. This sets the stage for a healthy microbiological ecosystem in the intestines. Besides the more common culprits known as the most prevalent food allergens, this also removes the "ultra-processed" or highly-processed food products in the diet because of the wide array of preservatives, hormones, antibiotics, or any other number of additives that may also pose unknown effects to digestive health. For the most part, it's best to avoid or minimize these types of highly processed "junk foods" that offer little-to-no nutritional value. This phase also removes irritants to the GI tract, such as too much alcohol, caffeine, or even certain medications. This includes a food elimination diet trial to determine which foods are part of the problem. Elimination diet trials primarily target the most common food allergens or other suspected causes of intolerances, such as gluten, dairy, corn, soy, eggs, shellfish, and sugar. An elimination diet trial may also incorporate a low FODMAP diet because many of the foods high in FODMAPs might help to explain food intolerances, yet might not be considered among the common food allergens. Remember, food allergies and food intolerances are different biological processes occurring in the body, yet are easily mistaken. The more strictly you follow this step, the more likely you are to find answers by noticing improvements in your symptoms and then identifying the problematic foods later, once you re-introduce them back into the diet one-by-one.

Sometimes this step only results in short-term relief, only to have the same problems eventually resurface. This may be a sign that the problematic gut bugs are hiding or protecting themselves underneath "biofilms." These biofilms that protect harmful bacteria are similar to how a house protects a family. This phase could require other products or treatments specifically to destroy these biofilms. It's only at this point, after addressing the underlying cause, that one can move on and effectively rebuild a balanced gut microbiome over time and a healthier lifestyle.

Phase 2 - Replace

This phase is about replacing some of the important factors required for normal digestive health that might be missing or inadequate. This can include not only the good gut bugs, but insufficient digestive enzymes, stomach acid, or even nutrients that one is deficient in. All of which are likely posing barriers to improved digestive function. Unfortunately, some of your good gut bugs, as well as the bad bacteria, that are part of the problem, will "die-off" due to the steps taken in Phase 1. This is why it's important to replace what was missing from your digestive tract before you rebuild or rebalance your gut ecosystem and proceed with a healthful diet.

We already recognized the importance of managing stress for normal digestion. Replacing multi-tasking at meals or mindless eating with mindfulness practices can be helpful to restore normal production of digestive enzymes. In other words, a state of chronic stress can impede the body's ability to produce digestive enzymes. A simple practice of stopping to say "thank you" (or a prayer) — whether to God, a higher power, or perhaps somebody you love or even a farmer that helped provide the food for you — before each meal, or practicing steps of mindful eating might help stimulate your initial phase of digestion. One culture that is known for incorporating this small but powerful practice of expressing gratitude before and after meals is the Japanese. In Japan people say "*itadakimasu*" before starting a meal and "*gochisousama*" after finishing the meal to show gratitude for nature and the people who brought the food to the table.[27] The initial phase of digestion helps keep the digestive enzymes flowing and promotes normal digestion after you eat a meal. Besides replacing missing factors like digestive enzymes or replacing distracted or mindless dining practices, like eating a meal while watching TV and scrolling through a cell phone app at the same time, this step is also about replacing unhealthful foods with nutrient-dense foods: that is, foods to provide nutrients, or building blocks, that the body and the brain demand to function optimally.

Phase 3 - Rebalance

When it comes to finding lasting relief from complex gut health disorders, fixing the problem of too many bad gut bugs is only the start of the journey. This third phase is also referred to as "Reinoculate" because it's about reintroducing or replanting your gut garden and then feeding your good gut bugs. This phase should include food sources of probiotics and prebiotics. Although there are still many unanswered questions about the safety and efficacy of supplements, this phase may or may not also include probiotics and/or prebiotics coming from dietary supplements (more on dietary supplements in Chapter 5). We also can't compare supplements to whole foods because of the synergistic effects of foods we don't quite understand. That is, we can't accurately measure just how important the naturally occurring and probiotic-created enzymes, vitamins, and other important "cofactors" (substances that aid the efficiency of chemical reactions in the body) from whole foods are to promoting overall health, let alone gut- and brain-health, in particular. Dietary supplements can be helpful for some but may not have as powerful, synergistic effects that whole foods tend to offer. Further, taking probiotics supplements at the wrong time for the wrong person might be more harmful than helpful. In general, it's best to focus more on food sources at this phase for most people.

When you repopulate your gut wall with healthy bacteria, this "reinoculation" of good gut bugs can help rebuild or strengthen your immune system. Research has shown that by increasing levels of certain bacteria populated in the gut, such as bifidobacterium (commonly found in various fermented foods, especially dairy), by modifying the diet may help reduce intestinal permeability (IP) as well as help lower inflammation[28].

Phase 4 - Repair

This phase is about repairing any damage to the intestinal cells (enterocytes and tight junctions that keep a seal between them) that may have occurred in the past. This also helps to tighten the seal between intestinal cells. Once the integrity of the gut-barrier is restored in this final step, then a robust and diverse gut microbiome provides an extra layer of protection and helps with normal digestion and immune system function. Certain nutrients are critical to the health and function of these intestinal cells.

Obtaining a sufficient intake of all the essential nutrients from the foods one eats can be very difficult and maybe even unrealistic for many people. Certain supplements may prove helpful for repairing a compromised gut-barrier. Unfortunately, however, there's no one-size-fits-all recommendation or regimen for dietary supplements to help with gut healing. One study published in 2019 aimed to investigate the most common and potentially beneficial supplements used among complementary and integrative medicine (CIM) practitioners. The researchers found that among the 36 Australian CIM practitioners included in the study, the most commonly used dietary supplements for treating increased intestinal permeability (IP; leaky gut) were zinc, vitamin D, glutamine, turmeric, "S. Boulardii" (probiotic, a strain of yeast) and multi-strain probiotics.[29] However, a couple of noteworthy remarks about this study. First, most of the CIM practitioners that successfully helped people resolve increased IP used multiple and diverse supplements and recommended reducing intakes of alcohol, gluten, and dairy. Also, the minimum amount of time required to resolve the IP was three months, some not seeing resolution until six months or longer. Understand that this is a process that requires patience. This process may even require a team of healthcare professionals, or for you to establish a support network of professionals who have troubleshot similar problems in the past.

CHAPTER 5

INTERMITTENT FASTING, KETOGENIC DIET, AND SUPPLEMENTS – HELPFUL OR HURTFUL?

Readers who have heard about intermittent fasting, ketogenic diets and supplements may be wondering about their potential benefits and risks. There's no one best diet that will work for all people. Nor is there a single diet that is compliant with a wide variety of dietary restrictions or religious or cultural preferences. Dietary needs and preferences are influenced by a variety of factors, such as pre-existing digestive problems, genetic and cultural backgrounds, just to name a few. In this chapter I'll discuss a few approaches to weight management and digestive disorders.

INTERMITTENT FASTING

With roots dating back to ancient times, fasting is a practice of refraining from eating any food for an extended period of time. There are quite a variety of reasons why one might choose to practice a fasting regimen. Whether for religious or spiritual practices, intended healing purposes, political causes such as peaceful protests and civil disobedience, or for expected health benefits and longevity. Fasting is and long has been a common practice around the world. Because fasting can also have unintended and potentially harmful health consequences, we must also discuss some possible disadvantages and limitations in the research. We'll also discuss how a more structured practice of fasting may have the potential to improve overall health. In particular, how a fasting regimen may help improve blood sugar control and digestion and support weight loss; and when followed in an informed manner, may even contribute to overall gut health and mental well-being.

Intermittent fasting (IF) is a term that is broadly used to describe a specified schedule of splitting waking hours between periods of eating hours and non-eating hours. There is no right or wrong way to practice IF. For example, people may restrict their "eating window" (time range which all calories are consumed) to an 8-hour window or to a 4-hour window one or two days weekly. This is one example of a form of fasting considered time-restricted feeding.[1] Some choose to do this more frequently such as restricting meals like this on a daily basis. However, I advise caution to anybody adopting a fasting regimen this way. Restricting your food on a daily basis limits your intake of important vitamins and minerals and may open the door to other problems with food like developing unhealthy thought patterns, disordered eating, or eventually for some, eating disorders such as anorexia or bulimia.

Others might fast for 24 hours once or twice monthly. A different approach towards fasting could have a modified schedule where one eats normally five days per week and then limits their food intake on two consecutive days on the weekend to less than or equal to 25% of estimated energy needs. Although there is no "best" regimen to practice IF, there are some things to consider and different models that can be followed in a more informed manner. Over time people practicing IF should modify their regimen depending on how they feel during fasting and on the intended and achieved outcomes.

Advantages and disadvantages of intermittent fasting

First, take this section with a bit of discretion because what's helpful for one person is not always helpful to another person when making dietary changes or following and adjusting to different eating patterns or schedules. The majority of the research findings on IF that suggest health benefits have been conducted on rodents. The limited research on humans is mostly based on observational research, and so we cannot determine cause and effect relationships from these types of research studies. In these observational studies researchers commonly collect evidence from a community of people fasting for religious purposes such as for Ramadan, an annual month-long practice of IF to honor Islamic beliefs. This disproportionate inclusion of a particular population in the studies available on IF is not necessarily representative of the general population. Also noteworthy are the small sample sizes of many of these observational human studies done on IF.

To better determine cause and effect relationships, we need more controlled and rigorous study designs, such as randomized controlled trials (RCTs), which are considered the gold standard for determining cause and effect relationships in science. We need more RCTs conducted with human participants and adequately sized sample populations. Further, RCTs should be followed by additional studies that yield comparable results (findings should be replicated) and help solidify our understanding of such complex topics in science. This is the direction of current research to further advance our understanding of the potential health advantages or disadvantages of practicing IF.

Advantages - Many purported, little substantiated, to be further researched

Some of the commonly purported benefits of fasting include improved blood sugar regulation, weight loss, digestive health, immune health, and even delaying the normal aging process. Extended periods of time between normal digestive processes allow the body to use energy for other processes such as repairing and healing from oxidative stress, cellular damage, and removal of a buildup of toxins.[2] One way to think of fasting is giving the metabolism a break from its normal functioning of digestive processes that typically occur around the clock. Therefore, structured practice of IF may be particularly beneficial for metabolic disorders, such as those with obesity trying to lose weight, manage diabetes, or may even potentially help prevent diabetes from developing.

One explanation of how IF can help impact blood sugar and weight management is by improving insulin sensitivity. Insulin sensitivity is a measure of how cell receptors respond to the presence of insulin, which is required for cells to permit blood sugar into the cells to provide energy. When the body is regularly exposed to higher levels of blood sugar from eating large portions of carbohydrate-containing foods, especially the refined types of foods low in fiber, this can lead to reduced insulin sensitivity or a down-regulation of the number of insulin receptors available on the cells. One way to think of insulin and cell receptor sites is like a keycard required for entry into a locked parking garage. If insulin is required for blood sugar to be allowed entry into the cells (and prevent excess sugar from circulating in the blood), then insulin receptors on cell surfaces are similar to the locked entryway into the parking garage and the insulin is the "keycard" required for entry. If there aren't enough entryways outside of the garage to permit cars into the garage, the cars might pile up and wait around without access, regardless of how many keycards are available. This is similar to how the body responds to regular high blood sugars. The receptors are no longer as sensitive and not as ready to permit glucose into the working cells to supply energy. Although there might be plenty of insulin available (assuming type 2 diabetes, and the pancreas still functions properly), insulin receptors can become less sensitive and less responsive to the circulating blood sugar that needs access or "entry" into the working cells.

Prolonged periods of fasting decrease insulin levels and in turn may improve sensitivity to glucose metabolism. Although this effect has been demonstrated in animal studies, the evidence of lasting effects of improved insulin sensitivity is less conclusive in human studies and so more studies need to be conducted before having adequate evidence to recommend IF (intermittent fasting) protocols for this purpose to the general public.[3] Additionally, of the human studies investigating IF and the effects on insulin resistance, many of these are of short duration, have few research participants, and have mixed findings. So it's difficult to conclude there is a body of definitive evidence from research conducted on humans with respect to IF.

For some, IF offers more flexibility towards dieting and weight loss. More traditional forms of dieting encourage chronic restriction of calories, where daily food intake is limited to approximately 20-40% less than normal intake. IF offers a different, more varied approach towards dieting with limited caloric intake. With IF, food intake is only restricted on certain days, while other days dietary intake is not changed. Many people see this as a more flexible approach towards trying to lose weight.[4] However, due to the shortage of research on the long-term effects of fasting, IF should not yet be recommended as a long-term solution to weight loss but may prove helpful to some in their weight loss journey, particularly in the short-term.

Regarding IF and potential benefits to digestive health and a normal functioning immune system, this matter is less well understood but seems to bring us right back to the importance of a balanced gut microbiome. Although the science is limited here, the mechanisms by which IF might help to reset an unbalanced gut microbiome — and therefore improve digestion and eventually immune health —are likely explained by longer durations of time between digestive processes and the disruption of the "normal feeding cycle" that typically provides a regular supply of carbohydrate-containing foods to the gut bugs. Over time, IF may have the effect of "starving off" some of the bad gut bugs and decreasing their population in the gut. In a sense, providing a cleaner slate to rebuild your microbial community with the foods you'll eat after IF. Granted, this is more theoretical than proven by science at this point. However, there's potential here to be further researched. In the future, we're likely to better understand how a regular and informed practice of IF may improve digestive problems for some people.

Now, the link between digestive health and immune health is more clear. Once chronic digestive issues are resolved, this tends to give way to improved immune health (not always the case). When the gut is given more time to rest it can help decrease intestinal permeability and inflammation. After improving digestion and cooling the fires of chronic inflammation through healthy diet and lifestyle changes, it's more likely that an overstimulated immune system can now get a break from its usual course of overworking. As you can see by now, this all connects to immune health and a proper functioning digestive system. For some people, you might consider IF one more tool in your toolbox as you practice lifestyle changes in your journey towards improving health. As to how much IF may or may not help those addressing digestive problems frankly remains unclear.

On such claims of "delaying the aging process" or "improved mental clarity", the potential here is likely attributed to the change of biological processes that occur during periods of fasting. Giving the body extended breaks from its normal cycle of digestion allows the body more time and ability to clean up cellular debris and waste that normally occur from daily stressors and throughout life. The limited research on this link mostly consists of animal-based studies. However, this research helps us understand ways in which a regular practice of IF may protect against damage to DNA. It is this normal, gradual process of degrading the protective features of our DNA that we largely attribute to the natural processes of aging. Similar to how regular exercise can promote enhanced neurogenesis (growth and development of the nervous system, including brain cells), restricting overall energy intake such as a practice of IF may also promote enhanced brain function.[5] Although this research is too early for us to recommend a practice of IF based on such tenuous claims, it is nonetheless exciting to think of the potential IF holds to impact one's metabolism, overall health, and longevity.

Disadvantages: Not Advised to Some, Caution to Others

When not practiced in a safe and informed manner, fasting can have concerning effects, such as fatigue, hunger, weakness, decreased alertness or trouble concentrating, and even dizziness.[6]

Some of these concerns are especially important for anybody with a history of diabetes, eating disorders, or being underweight. For those who have diabetes and are on insulin or other blood-sugar-lowering medications, fasting can be especially dangerous if not monitored correctly. This is particularly true for those who are at high risk for or regularly experience episodes of low blood sugar (hypoglycemia). Understand that diabetes is a metabolic disorder that is the result of dysregulation of a normal blood sugar balance. Going extended periods of time without food can further contribute to this dysregulation of blood sugar when the pancreas and insulin receptors do not function correctly, as is the case for people who have diabetes. Those with diabetes, hypertension, or heart disease and are on medications should make sure to be closely monitored by a doctor if they would like to consider practicing IF.

Fasting is not a good idea for those who have certain hypermetabolic conditions (significantly elevated needs for calories, proteins, and other nutrients) such as cancer, recovering from surgery or traumatic injuries like second or third-degree burns, or certain pulmonary conditions, such as chronic obstructive pulmonary disease or cystic fibrosis. Aside from these medical issues, the ones mentioned above and other hypermetabolic conditions, fasting is not recommended to children, adolescents, or women who are pregnant or breastfeeding. IF is also not recommended for those who recently had organ transplantation or others who have a compromised immune system.

Furthermore, prolonged periods of fasting can contribute to increased levels of the stress hormone, cortisol. Increased levels of cortisol can also promote weight gain. This should be taken into consideration if you already experience high-stress levels before starting a fasting regimen, especially for those trying to lose weight.

So, the potential benefits (or disadvantages) for weight loss that result from following a fasting regimen are not very clear. To reiterate, too rigid of an approach towards a practice of fasting can be a slippery slope to developing an unhealthy relationship with food (if one does not already exist). For example, if a person is disappointed in themselves for breaking a fast earlier than planned, they might become more inclined to have self-doubt, shame, or even feel guilty for not following their intended plan. These self-critical thoughts might be a sign of disordered eating and should be taken seriously if someone is beginning to think like this after starting to practice intermittent fasting. The bottom line here is that first and foremost, we need to regularly fuel ourselves with wholesome and nutritious foods and try not to follow too rigid rules when practicing fasting, which can ultimately contribute to more harm than benefit.

DIFFERENT MODELS OF FASTING

Similar to how there's no one-size-fits-all approach for the best dietary pattern, there's no best model of fasting that will work well for all people and different lifestyles. Let's not forget the importance of gradually working up to longer periods of fasting such as 24 hours or longer. Also, remember that it's okay if you set your mind on fasting for a certain amount of time and end up not feeling well or have unexpected symptoms and break the fast early. It may take time and practice until you feel more comfortable with fasting. Some models are more restrictive or even extreme than others, so use caution and be aware of this. A few of the more common IF models are described below.

16:8 Model

This model requires all food intake to be restricted to an 8-hour window. The period of sleeping would be included in the 16 hours that food is not ingested. People following this model typically do not eat for about eight hours after waking or for the last eight hours before bed.[7]

Although this model may sound relatively simple, in practice it may not be so easy for some to follow. Without gradually working up to such periods of fasting, simply avoiding foods for eight hours in the morning or for the last hours of being awake, may have unintended effects on sleep and mood.

5:2 Diet

Fast on two days per week and "eat normally" the other five days per week. For some following this pattern, it encourages eating whatever foods without much regard to ensuring an adequate intake of balanced food groups on the five non-fasting days. On the two days of fasting, food intake is restricted to approximately 25% of normal caloric needs. For example, if a person usually eats 2,000 calories per day, they would restrict food intake to about 500 calories per day on two days per week. When followed more strictly, however, this diet instructs to eat a "normal healthy Mediterranean style" diet on the five non-fasting days. This can also be considered a means of caloric restriction and potentially contribute to weight loss. The 5:2 method was developed by Dr. Michael Mosley and is also referred to as the Blood Sugar Diet.[8]

Eat, Stop, Eat: 24-hour fast, one to two times weekly

This method of IF includes practicing a 24-hour fast on one or two days weekly. First described by Brad Pilon, who has a background in the dietary supplement industry and developed this method after conducting graduate research in nutrition science.[9] This method is also a means of caloric restriction, though it may be relatively difficult to follow for those beginning a fasting regimen due to some of the reasons already discussed.

Alternate day fasting

Caution is advised here as this can be considered more extreme; it is minimally researched, potentially harmful, and perhaps unrealistic for most people. The alternate-day fasting method entails alternating between days restricting caloric intake to about 25% of usual intake and "feast days" where one ingests up to 125% of normal caloric intake. One randomized controlled trial published in 2017 found a high dropout rate in the group following an alternate day fasting method, suggesting that despite potential contributions to a caloric deficit and weight loss, this method may simply prove too uncomfortable or impractical for many people.[10]

Fasting-Mimicking Diet

In more recent years, various models of fasting have become more flexible. This is often a matter of making them appealing or realistic for a broader audience. Some of these are referred to as fasting-mimicking diets (FMD). One example of an FMD is seen in an experimental research study published in 2017 by Min Wei and fellow researchers at University of California, Los Angeles.[11] Wei and colleagues followed a regimen where people restricted their food intake for 5 consecutive days — approximately 40% of their usual caloric intake — each month for three consecutive months. Compared to those following a normal diet, this relatively permissive approach towards IF resulted in statistically significant improvements in body weight, total body fat, blood pressure, and insulin-like growth factor-1. This study from Wei and colleagues serves as a demonstration to the potential of fasting regimens to have an impact on metabolism, weight maintenance, and even mental well-being, most likely due to the link between IF and its impact on the microbiome and overall digestion.

BEFORE YOU BEGIN FASTING

Before you begin any type of IF regimen, run this decision by your doctor just to make sure you do not have any health conditions that might make fasting unsafe for you. Besides the other medical conditions discussed above, this is especially important for those with diabetes and who are taking medications for this condition. Fasting may result in dangerously low blood sugars in those with diabetes and so be sure to discuss this in detail if you have diabetes or have a history of diabetes or prediabetes or any of the other medical conditions discussed above. These may be indications you're not a good candidate for practicing an IF regimen.

Also, remember that it's important to drink water while fasting as you still need to stay hydrated. The human body can safely go much longer periods without food than without water. Lesser amounts of black coffee and tea are okay, but make sure to drink plenty of water first while fasting. If you have any other fluids, such as coffee or herbal teas, do not add any cream, sugar, or any other sweeteners that contribute calories to the fluids and could cause a spike in blood sugar and insulin. The bottom line is that there's still a lot we don't fully understand about the potential benefits or harm from a regular practice of fasting. So, do proper research first, work closely with your doctor, and start gradually. Perhaps just as important is to keep an open mind, have patience, and be flexible in your plans before beginning any fasting regimen.

One other result from a state of prolonged fasting is that the body reaches a state of ketosis. When the body reaches "ketosis" it means that the biochemistry of the body switches from using carbohydrates (glucose) as the primary source of energy to producing ketone bodies that become a primary source of energy to the body's working cells. This phenomenon is also what happens when people strictly follow extremely low carbohydrate diets. This leads to the next section about the ketogenic diet and why it has become so popular in recent years. Moreover, let's acknowledge the potential utility these diets (both intermittent fasting and ketogenic diet) can have for some people seeking not only weight improvement in general, but improved digestion and mental well-being, since these factors are so strongly related.

KETOGENIC DIET

Simply put, the ketogenic diet consists of following a very low-carbohydrate (approximately 25-50 grams carbohydrates per day) and a high-fat diet that provides adequate, not excessive protein. The ketogenic diet was developed 100 years ago and the original purpose had nothing to do with more common reasons many people tend to follow it nowadays. Historically, the one clinical indication for a prescribed ketogenic diet was for unmanageable epileptic seizures, particularly in children who had not achieved much relief through the help of medications. More recently the ketogenic or "keto diet" has gained a lot of popularity in the past couple of decades for other proclaimed reasons.[12] It's these other more recently purported benefits we must explore briefly, considering that following this diet may also have effects (potentially beneficial or harmful) and impact your mental well-being along your journey of making lifestyle changes.

The keto diet greatly contrasts with what most healthy dietary patterns recommend. As previously discussed, most experts agree that a balanced diet includes a variety of fruits, vegetables, whole grains, and legumes (beans, lentils, peas, etc.). The keto diet limits or restricts many of these healthy fiber-containing foods and, therefore, is often accompanied by some undesirable side effects, especially when not followed in an informed manner. Considering this departure from a generally accepted healthful diet, the keto diet is not recommended long-term, for either weight loss or blood sugar control. Although the benefits of following a keto diet for those suffering from intractable epilepsy (uncontrolled by medications) potentially outweigh long-term health consequences or side effects, it's not this population we need to discuss in this book.

UNANSWERED QUESTIONS - SHORT-TERM BENEFITS VS. LONG-TERM COSTS

Potential benefits: Short-term vs. long-term

Despite the many uncertainties or unanswered questions in research, many people experience impressive short-term weight loss results from following a ketogenic diet. Also, the positive effects on blood sugar regulation are commonly reported. This suggests the potential for people with diabetes to better manage blood sugar levels. For many people, short-term progress can be exciting, motivating, and promote personal convictions about following such a dietary pattern. However, these fast-achieved results don't take into consideration potential long-term costs or concerns that we don't yet have a thorough understanding of.

Most of the weight loss from following any low-carbohydrate diet in the first couple of days to weeks is due to the body burning up stored carbohydrates in the liver and muscles. These stored carbohydrates (glycogen) also hold onto water. Hence, much of the weight loss people experience in the first couple weeks of a low carbohydrate diet is the body burning up the stored glycogen and the water weight being released. Therefore, initial results from following any carbohydrate-restricted diet are not necessarily as much from fat loss, as people anticipate, but from following such a restrictive diet.

The rapid weight loss achieved following a low carb diet is often short-term and people are likely to regain much of the weight as fast as it was lost once they reintroduce a more normal amount of carbohydrates into the diet. Or, perhaps, frustration sets in from abstaining from too many foods and then feeling deprived. For some, this sense of deprivation might contribute to binge-eating lower quality, highly refined carbohydrate foods (e.g., cookies, chips, cakes, and candies). This does not help with maintaining a sustainable, healthy relationship with food. Furthermore, regularly going from one drastic dietary change to another is not a good thing for health.

However, some people do follow a low-carb or ketogenic diet for longer periods of time, sometimes with more lasting results. Besides shifting to dietary fat as a primary source of energy (compared to using more carbohydrates as a primary source), the ketogenic diet can contribute to weight loss by helping suppress appetite and regulating hunger hormones, increasing the energy required to metabolize foods, and better control of insulin which limits storage of dietary fat.[13] Gibson and colleagues conducted a systematic review and meta-analysis (results compiled from multiple studies) to investigate the effects of a calorie-restricted ketogenic diet on hunger levels. They concluded that there's a significant correlation between following a ketogenic diet and reduced hunger levels.[14]

Although people with obesity following a calorie-restricted diet typically report increased hunger levels, following a ketogenic diet may prove helpful to some trying to lose weight and struggling with hunger levels and not feeling full (low satiety). Also, given that carbohydrates stimulate insulin release and high insulin levels prevent the breakdown of stored body fat, following a low-carbohydrate diet reduces insulin. This can help the body become more efficient at burning stored fat as a vast supply of energy needs.

Concerns and Potential Costs: Short-term vs. Long-term

As the body adjusts to a carbohydrate-restricted diet many people experience what's commonly referred as the "keto flu", mostly occurring in the first week or two. Note that the "keto flu" is not a recognized medical condition and is not the same as the flu virus that infects many people regardless of their dietary intake. Rather, it's a term used to describe the cluster of symptoms commonly experienced in the early stages of following a ketogenic diet. These symptoms include "headache, fatigue, irritability, nausea, difficulty sleeping, and constipation", just to name a few.[15] In the first couple of days to the first couple weeks, other common side effects include low blood sugar, dizziness, vomiting, diarrhea, gastroesophageal reflux (GERD), and metabolic acidosis.[16]

Unfortunately, we don't have a clear understanding of what causes this common cluster of symptoms. Some of the unpleasant symptoms might be related to loss of electrolytes and dehydration, which can result in fatigue and general weakness. Therefore, it's important to drink plenty of fluids and sometimes people need a little extra intake of foods high in electrolytes, such as sodium, potassium, and magnesium. If left untreated, electrolyte imbalances could even cause kidney injury or heart arrhythmias (abnormal rhythm). The phenomenon referred to as the "keto flu" typically only lasts about a week (some report this for up to a month) and is more of a short-term concern. After following a relatively healthy ketogenic diet for a week or two, most cells in the body have shifted to using fatty acids as the preferred source of energy rather than glucose, and the brain and nervous system cells are utilizing fat indirectly through the production of ketones.[17] Many people tend to report feeling much better after getting past this point in the diet.

Also noteworthy is the rigidness and necessity for attention to detail to follow the ketogenic diet. This in and of itself might prove unrealistic or unappealing for most people. As mentioned, too much protein can prevent the body from going into ketosis and not achieving desired results. However, inadequate protein intake (not as likely as excessive protein) along with a calorie-restricted diet can also result in feeling weak and listless, and more prone to getting sick from an impaired immune system. Furthermore, there is a desired range of ketones in the body chemistry required in order to achieve optimal results. This level of "ketosis" can be tested by urine test strips (purchased at local drug stores) or by a blood test ordered by a doctor. Although testing via urine strips is cheaper and easier, it's considered less accurate than the blood test.

Having too high levels of ketones can be harmful to some people. This is particularly important for those who have pre-existing metabolic disorders such as diabetes. Having excessive blood ketones is considered ketoacidosis, more commonly seen in people with diabetes, referred to as diabetic ketoacidosis. When not treated, this can be very dangerous and include a variety of symptoms or even result in coma or death. Ketoacidosis can also be especially harmful to people who have pancreatitis or kidney disease.

Considering the long-term effects of following a ketogenic diet, this is an area that we still need more research on. Long-term studies are limited and inconsistent, and generally don't last longer than six months which limits our understanding of potential concerns that might arise after years of following a ketogenic diet. Due to this shortage of research on the long-term effects of the keto diet, I won't cover this in-depth here given that the limited scope makes it difficult to conclude much about long-term side effects. However, some of the potential long-term harm from following a ketogenic diet may include developing kidney stones, gallstones, constipation, or dehydration, just to name a few of the more probable issues. It's primarily for these reasons that the keto diet is not recommended as a long-term solution to weight loss, but may prove helpful for many in the short run when used strategically.

DIETARY SUPPLEMENTS

Therapeutic potential or potential for harm?

Let's consider two common concerns regarding dietary supplements in general. First, it can be difficult to determine the quality and effectiveness of various supplements. Regulation of the supplement industry by the Food and Drug Administration (FDA) is limited. A 1994 law speaks only to labeling and manufacturing of supplements.[18] It requires manufacturers to represent to the FDA that a product doesn't contain an unsafe or risky ingredient and is accurately labeled and to report any bad side effects consumers have experienced. Whereas a pharmaceutical manufacturer is required to submit a great deal of scientific evidence to the FDA that a particular drug is safe and effective before the FDA will grant permission to market and sell the drug, no such requirement exists for supplements. On the contrary, the FDA has to prove that a supplement is defective or unsafe before it can remove the product from the market.[19]

If you are looking for companies that are more likely to be trustworthy and reliable, one thing to look for is a symbol or logo that indicates the use of a third-party certification body or verification program. A third-party certification indicates that the company paid another company to test its products and verify the purity of its products. Some common third-party seals to look for are: ConsumerLab, NSF Certified for Sport, and USP Verified. Examples are shown in Figure 3 below.

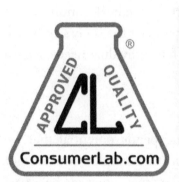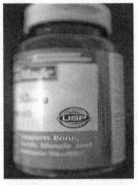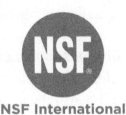

FIGURE 3. Examples of third-party certification symbols found on dietary supplements

Secondly, we have individual needs! People respond differently to diet changes and environmental and everyday stressors. There is no one-size-fits-all recommendation for taking dietary supplements with regard to improving mental well-being. Some people may greatly benefit from adopting a supplement regimen, while others might not realize any noticeable improvements. Or even worse, some people might be harmed from taking too much or taking supplements when not needed. So, make sure to do your homework and discuss your plans with your healthcare provider before adopting any supplement regimen.

Despite the potential for dietary supplements to improve nutritional inadequacies, complement existing treatments, and contribute to improved mental well-being, they do not take the place of eating a healthy diet. Just like the words suggest, dietary supplements are used to supplement one's diet. One common reason people use these products is to help fill the gaps of a nutritionally-deficient diet and supply more of the essential nutrients to achieve the recommended nutrient intakes. Supplements are also used to provide individual nutrients at higher doses than typically consumed in one's diet, for presumed health benefits. Another reason some find greater utility in taking supplements is that they can provide more bioavailable (readily available to the body after ingesting) forms. This may be particularly helpful for people that either have genetic predispositions to certain medical conditions or others with certain medical conditions that impact the body's ability to absorb nutrients. Everybody is unique and has individual needs, health concerns, and dietary preferences.

Role of supplements in mental health

Although supplements may have some therapeutic potential that we still don't fully understand, it must be noted that supplements are not *the* answer to fix mental health problems. They may, however, be a part of the solution for some people. In other words, when indicated certain dietary supplements may be one component of a more comprehensive treatment plan for treating mental illness. Also due to the minimal regulation and oversight in the supplement industry, there's inadequate evidence for most supplements to support standardization of dosages and recommendations, and, moreover, to prove the potential effectiveness of taking such supplements. So, much of the therapeutic potential for using supplements to improve mental well-being remains uncertain or in some cases, not readily accepted or understood in the medical community.

Published in 2019, Firth and colleagues advanced our understanding of the effectiveness of using dietary supplements as a complementary treatment to mental illness. Quite the comprehensive study, Firth compiled the results of 33 different meta-analyses of research about the safety and effectiveness of using supplements for treating mental illnesses. This meta-review represented the totality of the 33 different meta-analyses, some with inconsistent or inconclusive findings. Considering the safety or risks of taking supplements, this study found "no evidence of serious adverse effects or contraindications with psychiatric medications."[20] In all of the studies included in this meta-review, dietary supplements were taken simultaneously with "usual care", including common psychiatric medications.

Although there hasn't been adequate evidence to promote the widespread use of dietary supplements for complementing psychiatric treatment, recent evidence suggests the potential of certain dietary supplements to improve symptoms of depression in those who have deficient nutrient intakes. In those who are either deficient or have other reasons for elevated needs (such as impaired absorption), some of the key nutrients in the form of dietary supplements may prove helpful for improving mental health outcomes — omega-3s, various B-vitamins, essential minerals, magnesium, and zinc, and probiotics, just to name a few.

Omega-3 Fatty Acids

Among the most studied nutrients related to mental health outcomes, polyunsaturated fats (particularly omega-3s) have shown the potential to help improve symptoms of depression. Mostly attributed to the established link between chronic inflammation and major depression along with the anti-inflammatory properties of omega-3s, some experts propose omega-3 fatty acids as a potential treatment for major depression.[21]

There have, however, been mixed results in studies about the effectiveness of omega-3s for treating depression and, therefore, there is not yet a consensus among experts. When the researchers investigated these mixed results, they concluded that a higher ratio of EPA omega-3s to DHA omega-3s tended to result in more significant effects, particularly in study participants with major depressive disorder taking antidepressants. Hence, omega-3 supplementation may soon prove to be an effective complementary treatment to existing antidepressant medications. However, we must be mindful of the quality and reliability of the particular supplement brand and the potential long-term side effects (not well-researched) from taking high doses of omega-3 supplements for long periods of time.

B-vitamins

Folic acid (also referred to as vitamin B9, called folate in its food form)
There is some evidence that supplementing folic acid can enhance the effectiveness of depression medications in those with deficient levels of folate. Specifically, psychiatric meds referred to as "SSRIs"(selective serotonin reuptake inhibitors). Although there's not adequate evidence that supplementing folic acid alone (without SSRI treatment) can improve mood or depressive symptoms, this may improve depressive symptoms in conjunction with psychiatric medications.[22] People who are deficient in folate and taking antidepressants more commonly don't experience great results from the medication. A daily supplement of folic acid might enhance the effectiveness of SSRI medications for some people. If you and your healthcare provider decide that you might benefit from a folate supplement, keep in mind the recommended limit of 1,000 micrograms per day (for adults, even less for children/adolescents). If you supplement too much folic acid this can result in concealing a deficiency in B-12, which could cause other health problems similar to that of a folate deficiency.[23]

Vitamins B-6 and B-12

Besides folate, the evidence for the effects of other supplemental B-vitamins to improve mood is not as clear. However, because these nutrients are so important for a healthy nervous system and maintaining normal production of neurotransmitters that regulate our energy and mood, for some people it may not be a bad idea to consider a supplemental B-complex as part of a comprehensive plan.

Overall, the evidence for supplementing these other B-vitamins for improving mental health outcomes is just not as clear or as conclusive compared to what has been found among those taking folic acid supplements or some of the other nutrients discussed. Although the science is still mostly theoretical, one potential mechanism for how supplementation of folic acid, vitamins B-6, and B-12 might improve mental health outcomes has to do with the important roles they all serve in regulating levels of homocysteine in the body. Homocysteine is simply an amino acid, a natural byproduct of quite a variety of biochemical reactions in the body. When this particular amino acid builds up in the body without being further processed — likely the result of inadequate intakes of these important B-vitamins — this is related to increased chances of decreased blood flow, stroke, and unnecessary clotting of the blood.[24] Although it's natural to have levels of homocysteine increase in the blood as we age, these potentially life-threatening links associated with high homocysteine levels are perhaps a hallmark of overall cognitive decline as we age. This suggests that the link between very low levels of these B-vitamins and cognitive function may even have other detrimental effects on the nervous system and brain health.

B-vitamins are considered water-soluble. This means that they are dissolved in water (unlike fat-soluble vitamins, which store in fat cells) and are passed through the urine when we ingest too much of them. For most people in good health taking too much B-vitamin is not a health concern, just an unnecessary expense. However, there are some medical conditions with which a supplemental B-complex or high dose individual B-vitamins should not be taken. So make sure to run your plan by your medical provider prior to starting any supplemental regimen.

Given the relationship between folate and vitamin B-12, it's important to determine which one (or both) you are truly deficient in prior to starting a supplement regimen. This is because taking more of a folate supplement when you are not deficient in it, yet are deficient in B-12, can mask or hide the problems one might experience from a B-12 deficiency until problems have worsened.[25] This is the same for the other way around, — taking a B-12 supplement when a person is actually deficient in folate, can hide — or even worsen — some of the neurological symptoms related to the folate deficiency. For this reason and for many people, it's not a bad idea to supplement these nutrients together, such as in a B-complex supplement. Certain people are at a higher risk of deficient intakes of vitamin B-12 and may benefit from taking a supplement. Some populations are routinely recommended to supplement B-12 and other B-vitamins, specifically, vegetarians or vegans, or people who have had certain gastrointestinal surgeries (gastric bypass/weight loss surgery) or chronic inflammatory conditions of the gut such as Crohn's disease or celiac disease, which can affect absorption of nutrients, particularly B-12.

Magnesium

Earlier in this book, I explained how important magnesium is for overall health and for neurological health in particular. More broadly, magnesium is needed to help build and maintain a well-protected nervous system and to help you feel relaxed, though the evidence for using magnesium supplements for mental health disorders is just not clear or conclusive. In a systematic review of the research on this topic compiled by researchers in 2017, they concluded that evidence of benefit was inconsistent and limited, yet demonstrates the potential for helping some people improve subjective anxiety and stress levels.[26] Before these findings can be strengthened and magnesium subsequently recommended to the public to treat anxiety, we must conduct more high-quality randomized controlled trials in hopes to find more promising and informative results.

The research regarding magnesium supplementation and effects on depression is also a bit inconclusive, similar to what is found in studies among those with anxiety-related disorders. Despite the lack of evidence demonstrating how magnesium supplementation might help people with depression, some evidence does point specifically to its potential for improving symptoms of depression in those with treatment-resistant depression.[27] In other words, those who haven't found much relief from standard forms of treatment for depression may stand to benefit the most from the supplementation of magnesium. A review and meta-analysis in 2018 concluded that the benefits to mood reported after taking magnesium supplements were only found in uncontrolled studies, and no significant effect were found in the placebo-controlled studies.[28] This suggests that there may be a placebo effect on mood from taking a magnesium supplement.

Zinc

Similar to magnesium, researchers have long been exploring the link between low zinc levels and depression and the role this important trace mineral plays in neurological health more broadly. However, this link does not help us understand who may or may not improve their sense of mental well-being from taking a zinc supplement. In a scientific review from 2019, Basharat and colleagues examined seven different studies (five including human subjects, two including animals) investigating the role of zinc supplementation on improving depression. This review concluded that zinc supplementation may prove helpful in reducing the severity of symptoms of depression.[29] On the other hand, what proves helpful to some people is not always helpful to others when it comes to making dietary changes.

One note of caution is that there can be harmful consequences from taking too much of certain essential vitamins or minerals and zinc is one of these that can have unintended consequences. Considered a "trace mineral", zinc is important to include in the diet but in very small quantities. For example, if you take too much supplemental zinc this could result in a deficiency of copper, another important trace mineral in the diet.[30] For this reason, when taking a zinc supplement, it's usually a good idea to either limit the amount to the Recommended Dietary Intake or take supplemental copper simultaneously to reduce the likelihood of copper deficiency. Although the specific amounts of these supplements sometimes recommended are outside the scope of this book, it's important to illustrate this as one example of why you should not just start taking various supplements based on one research link. Or maybe even worse, you hear recommendations or testimonials of promising results from friends, family, celebrities, or others that take certain supplements and then you take this as proof of effectiveness and expect the same results.

Amino Acids

Amino acids are simply the building blocks of protein, provided from the foods eaten. Recall that these building blocks are not only for proteins that supply your muscles and vital organs, but they're also required to produce a steady supply of neurotransmitters that help regulate mood. A variety of amino acids are usually abundantly provided in the diet, however, many people don't eat a balanced diet and may also have other lifestyle factors that impact the body's production of neurotransmitters. For example, one theory suggests that eating a relatively low-carbohydrate/high-protein diet reduces the amount of tryptophan that is made available for the brain, relative to the other amino acids. This concept is referred to as the "Wurtman hypothesis" and suggests this competition with other amino acids in the bloodstream can limit the amount of tryptophan made available to produce serotonin.[31] Some believe that, in turn, this inadequate supply of tryptophan can contribute to the dysregulation of serotonin and consequently contribute to symptoms of depression.

There's some evidence that supplementation of certain key amino acids — particularly tryptophan — may prove helpful in improving the treatment of depression. Perhaps most commonly known and studied for several decades, tryptophan is an essential amino acid that is a building block required to produce melatonin (sleep-regulating hormone) and serotonin (mood-regulating neurotransmitter). These two key biological regulators help promote a normal sleep cycle as well as a normal, healthy mood. You might be thinking, can't we just eat more foods that are high in tryptophan? There is no solid evidence that levels of serotonin can be increased by eating more foods high in the amino acid tryptophan. This may be due to the "Wurtman hypothesis" discussed above, but it's not known with much certainty. If this hypothesis is accurate, then it's suggested that supplementation of certain amino acids such as tryptophan (commonly sold as 5-HTP) may help the body and brain utilize more of these key amino acids in people with inadequate levels of serotonin.

Other amino acids researched that show potential to improve mood include tyrosine, phenylalanine, and methionine.[32] We need further studies to determine what doses are effective and who may or may not benefit from such dietary supplementation.

Probiotics

By definition probiotics are "live microorganisms that, when administered in adequate amounts, confer a health benefit on the host."[33] However, the benefits of taking probiotics are dependent on the particular strain, the viability or quality of the product, and on the number of probiotics (referred to as colony-forming units). Furthermore, the right strain of bacteria needs to be matched with the particular condition or disease that is being targeted. In other words, "the efficacy of probiotic products is both strain-specific and disease-specific."[34] It wasn't until just a few years ago that researchers accumulated enough research to present an "evidence-based practical guide" for matching the correct strain of probiotic with the particular medical condition that evidence shows it may benefit.[35] This guide shows which strains have the strongest evidence for effectiveness and which ones have the weakest evidence and are, therefore, least likely to help. Although probiotic supplements may prove helpful for many — particularly for improving digestive issues like irritable bowel syndrome or antibiotic-associated diarrhea — it's not always a good idea to just start taking one without regard to any of the factors discussed above.

More directly relevant to mental health, a scientific review from 2016 examined the results of ten randomized controlled trials that studied the effects of probiotic supplementation on symptoms of anxiety and depression. Despite the limitations of this study, it did find limited evidence that supplementation can help improve reported symptoms of depression and anxiety. Of note, however, only four of the ten studies included in this review included people who were clinically diagnosed with depression or anxiety.[36] Given the many unanswered questions about which strains are required to help which people, we don't yet have strong enough evidence to conclude a one-size-fits-all recommendation for taking probiotics.

HELPFUL OR HURTFUL?
Not THE answer, but maybe ONE answer

For some in their journey towards healthful changes and improved mental well-being, this may include trials of intermittent fasting, a ketogenic diet, and/or a regimen of dietary supplements. For others, these may be of no importance depending on their situation. Each of these dietary options (intermittent fasting, ketogenic diet, and dietary supplements) require that you take into consideration your unique health conditions, concerns, and goals.

Although informative and practical science on intermittent fasting is still in its early days, some of the evidence is impressive and eventually may prove helpful at improving existing treatments for digestive conditions or metabolic disorders, such as diabetes and obesity. For some people, once they find relief for complex or previously unaddressed digestive disorders and improve chronic stress levels, this may give way to improved mental health outcomes.

Beyond the purpose of helping suppress the frequency of uncontrolled seizures, a closely monitored ketogenic diet can be followed in a relatively healthy manner. But remember it is important to make sure to get properly screened to determine if you're a good candidate prior to making such drastic dietary changes. For instance, those with kidney disease, diabetes, or other metabolic diseases should not follow a ketogenic diet without the close supervision of a skilled medical professional.

For those deemed a good candidate, a keto diet can prove helpful in the short-term for jumpstarting weight loss. Even more interesting, however, is how this diet — similar to intermittent fasting — may prove helpful when making dietary changes to address underlying digestive problems standing in the way to other general healthful changes. For example, people who have irritable bowel syndrome may not be able to tolerate a variety of healthy, high-fiber foods. They might see improvements in digestion from following a ketogenic diet and this can lead to more sustainable lifestyle changes, eventually giving way to improvements in mental well-being.

When followed in a more informed, "relatively healthful" and prescriptive manner, a ketogenic diet should include a variety of nourishing foods and not just regard the relative ratios of fats to carbs eaten at meals (as many programs may do). Considering the quality of fats and proteins, and the adequacy of dietary fiber, a proper keto diet should consist of plentiful colorful non-starchy vegetables and various sources of essential fats, such as nuts, seeds, fish, avocados, and olive oil. Instead of the factory-farmed meats sold in most fast-food restaurants and grocery stores, opt for more variety of protein foods like salmon, tuna, mahi mahi, scallops, and grass-fed beef products when available. Even sardines and anchovies are excellent choices for those brave enough! A ketogenic diet should include moderate amounts of varied protein sources. Ingesting too much protein can result in the body converting excess protein to blood glucose and not adhering to what is truly considered a ketogenic diet. In other words, too much protein prevents the body from staying in a state of ketosis and may prevent what keto dieters are trying to achieve.

The long-term effects of following a very low-carbohydrate, high fat diet aren't well understood, and might vary among different populations. Despite the exciting and often-achieved short-term results, one should also take into consideration potential long-term consequences from following a ketogenic diet for extended periods of time.[37] If you decide that following a ketogenic diet is right for you for a trial period, remember that it's important to be monitored by a skilled physician and a dietitian (and/or integrative & functional nutritionist) who has specialized training in ketogenic diets.

Similar to IF and the ketogenic diet, dietary supplements may play an important part in your journey towards lifestyle changes and improved health. Due to the precautions mentioned above for supplements as to personalized needs and the uncertainty among researchers, it is not my intention to offer a protocol. Rather, I want you to realize that the potential benefits of taking dietary supplements are very individualized. Some of these have drug-nutrient interactions with medications you may be taking, so you should always do additional research and discuss with your doctor prior to starting any particular supplement regimen.

PART III

CRAFTING YOUR FOODS FOR THOUGHT GAME PLAN

A goal without a plan is just a wish.

ANTOINE DE SAINT-EXUPERY

CHAPTER 6

FORGET DIETS: THREE GUIDING PRINCIPLES

Let's understand that everybody makes changes at their own pace and that it's alright to eat some processed foods. Just because a food is processed does not mean it is "bad" or inherently unhealthy. Likewise, some foods that are considered healthy eaten in low-moderate amounts may not be considered healthy when eaten in large quantities, or can even contribute to the development of chronic diseases. Many healthy food staples are processed as a means to extend the shelf life and reduce waste or modify the consistency and taste to varied palates and needs of consumers. Some of these food staples can include whole-grain (low-sugar) cereals, applesauce, or even guacamole, just to name a few. Although the processing of foods may alter the nutritional value, it does not completely devalue the nutritional worth of eating these foods. More importantly, the degree of processing should be taken into consideration because various cooking and processing methods can deplete certain nutrients, whereas other minimally processed food products may have been produced under standards that better preserved the nutritional value of the food.

Consider how extra virgin olive oil is a nutritionally-superior product to the average, cheaper refined olive oil which is subjected to higher heat through processing. The high-heat, along with various chemicals used in processing, results in a product with less of the protective antioxidants and can alter the healthfulness of the important unsaturated fats that occur naturally in the olives, but with a more stable and longer-lasting "shelf-life." This is but one example of how various degrees of food processing can alter the healthful properties of certain foods. This example of devaluing the nutritional value of food through processing serves to help you appreciate how eating a diet filled with mostly processed foods and food products can be a major contributor to nutritional deficiencies. And perhaps more importantly, this "standard American diet" could be a predominant contributing factor to most health problems that plague the U.S., including physical and mental health.

But even small amounts of what some refer to as "ultra-processed foods" or "food-like substances" are fine to eat in moderation for most people. There are a few exceptions for certain ingredients (found in many of these highly processed products) for people with certain conditions, such as food allergies or intolerances, as well as people following an elimination diet trial to help determine what are some of the problematic "trigger foods" likely contributing to unknown food allergies, intolerances, or other gastrointestinal problems. Some examples of these products found in most grocery stores include (not limited to) cupcakes, candy bars, high-sugar cereals, various white breads, and flour-based bakery goods and pastries, or processed cheeses and meats such as can-squeezed cheese, hot dogs, pepperoni, sausage, bologna, etc. For simplicity's sake, we will broadly refer to all of these foods — and many more like these — as *highly processed food products (HPFPs)*.

Overall, however, it is a good rule of thumb to either avoid or minimize the intake of these HPFPs and first fill up on whole foods, mostly plant-based. Or better yet, when you want the occasional indulgent sweet and/or salty treat, why not practice making your own using healthier ingredients and have control over how much of each ingredient is used. This leaves the option of modifying recipes to make them healthier than standard favorites found in your local grocery stores and restaurants. So we'll explore different model dietary patterns that first load up on whole foods, mostly plant-based. After making diet changes over longer periods of time, once your diet is "crowded out"[1] with a variety of nutrient-dense whole-foods, then the occasional sweet treat, salty fried snack, or whatever other highly processed food you choose is perfectly fine to eat in moderation. Keyword: moderation.

In this chapter I'll discuss some of the most important principles to keep in mind, regardless of which dietary pattern you might decide to follow. In other words, this chapter will help you understand what constitutes an optimal diet for overall health —one that contributes to digestive and brain health —so that you can begin to craft your own *Foods for Thought Game Plan*.

PRINCIPLE 1:
DIETS DO NOT WORK: IT'S THE PATTERN THAT MATTERS

When I say "forget diets" or "diets do not work" I am referring to fad diets that promise miracle cures or magical weight loss, not diets recommended by registered dietitians, complementary and integrative medicine practitioners or physicians to treat troubling symptoms and diagnosed diseases. For most people, rather than looking for a quick-fix diet, it's important to think about what you typically eat — in other words, your eating pattern. Some important questions to consider: How many servings of fruits and vegetables do you eat per day on an average week? How many servings of whole grains and legumes do you eat per week? Are most of the sources of carbohydrates you eat coming from refined grains and added sugars with little nutritional value? Do you eat a variety of lean proteins, including animal-based and plant-based proteins? How often do you eat processed meats? Do you eat too many processed oils and fried foods, and not enough sources of essential, unsaturated fats?

These questions help you reflect on where your biggest areas for improvement are when establishing a plan and adopting lifestyle changes. These questions are about the pattern of your diet. Because there is no one-size-fits-all diet that appeals or works well for all people, identifying your key areas for improvement on diet and lifestyle changes will help you find an individualized pathway to making lifestyle changes (however imperfectly and at your own pace) for the rest of your life, to benefit your health and quality of life. As you can probably tell by now, this book is not about following a diet.

If you have tried different diets multiple times in the past with certain food groups restricted or avoided, this restriction is part of the reason why these diets are not sustainable, realistic or sometimes can even be harmful for people to follow. Despite the often achieved short-term and impressive results from following some of these diets, these are not long-term solutions to health problems that likely developed over long periods of time. This is also partly why so many people fail on diets. Nobody wants to be stuck with feelings of being deprived, hungry, or having constant cravings for certain forbidden foods.

Further, health problems such as obesity, depression, and anxiety are complex. Following rigid diet plans may result in seemingly promising short-term results —particularly for weight loss attempts or blood sugar control — though without acknowledging potential long-term costs of following restrictive-type diets, you could be posing more harm in the long run. For sustainable success, you must take a realistic and individualized approach towards your own health journey. Find what works for you, find what does not work, and over time you can modify and refine your *Foods for Thought Game Plan*. Another person's diet or lifestyle plan— whether a friend, family member, or even recommended by a celebrity — may not be your best fit.

COMPARING HEALTHY PATTERNS — LESSONS FROM THE BLUE ZONES

There is a great variety of contrasting dietary patterns among different cultures around the world. This speaks to the amazing ability of the human body to adapt to a wide range of different dietary intakes and still meet basic nutrition needs. One award-winning book that beautifully illustrates this range of diverse diets is *Hungry Planet: What the World Eats*.[2] Traditional diets vary considerably with emphasis on different food groups but the lesson here is that there are options of dietary patterns or models to follow that can be considered healthy and contribute to overall gut health, and therefore brain health. Despite all of the confusing research often cited in the media and unsettled questions in nutrition science about what constitutes an optimal diet for human health, let's focus more on what researchers and experts can generally all agree on.

First, look at the dietary commonalities of what can be considered among the healthiest populations in the world. Perhaps it makes sense to take lessons from certain populations around the world who notably live past 100 years old in better health, compared to other developed regions of the world with normal life expectancies. These populations are recognized as the Blue Zones, identified by Dan Buettner and his team of researchers along with the help of colleagues at the National Geographic and the National Institute on Aging.[3] These regions are: Icaria (Greece), Loma Linda (California, U.S.), Nicoya (Costa Rica), Okinawa (Japan), and Sardinia (Italy).

Citizens in these five regions are known for their remarkably healthy and socially connected lifestyles, which contribute to their longer than usual life spans and, possibly, to their lower levels of dementia and depression. Based on this evidence, one might easily assume that people living in these Blue Zones must be following an optimally healthy diet that promotes good brain health and longevity. Compared to those eating a standard American diet (SAD), those in Blue Zones tend to eat greater amounts of whole foods, mostly plant-based. This means more fruits, vegetables, legumes (beans, lentils, peas, and soybeans/tofu), and whole grains in their minimally processed forms. Unlike most Americans, these populations eat meat in moderation, if at all. In four of the five Blue Zones it is more common to eat meat sparingly, such as one 3-5-ounce portion one time weekly. Regular and moderate consumption of alcohol (1-2 drinks per day, preferably red wine) is common in these populations. In Loma Linda, members of a community of nearly 10,000 Seventh Day Adventists predominantly eat a vegetarian diet and abstain from meat and alcohol, mostly choosing a whole foods plant-based diet instead.

Remember, this is not all about diet and food choices. Those living in the Blue Zones also tend to have healthy lifestyle patterns. Let's not give all the credit for good health and longevity of these populations to eating a healthy diet. Given the importance of other lifestyle factors for promoting mental well-being, we must recognize other factors contributing to the exceptional health of inhabitants of the Blue Zones.

Referred to as the Power 9, there are nine principles or common characteristics found among these regions.[4] Similar to the concepts about wellness and self-care discussed in the Afterword, the Power 9 encompasses other aspects of overall health, such as being socially and spiritually connected, having a positive mental outlook and better destressing from everyday stressors. Contrary to general healthful exercise recommendations in the U.S., these populations tend to opt for natural daily movement, such as maintaining gardens or walking as a means of transportation, and for doing daily chores. For a detailed look at the Power 9, visit Bluezones.com.

PRINCIPLE 2:
TOO MUCH OF A GOOD THING IS NOT SO GOOD

Let's not forget the importance of temperance. In contrast with people who consume the "standard American diet", those living in the Blue Zones promote a sense of balance and do not overindulge on any particular food or food group. Commonly, people tend to think of individual foods in terms of either being "good" or "bad." Not only does this oversimplified, reductionist mindset toward the healthfulness of foods confuse most consumers but it also obscures the *more important* concept of following a healthy eating pattern. However, there are certain foods that can be part of a healthy eating pattern but when eaten in excess, over time may be harmful and significantly increase one's chances of developing various chronic diseases that claim the lives of most Americans.

There is a body of research demonstrating the significant relationship between the amount of animal-based proteins a person eats and the chances of getting cancer. In other words, limited amounts of meat and dairy can help meet your nutrition needs and can be part of a healthy diet, whereas regularly eating large amounts of these animal-based proteins in excess of estimated protein needs has been linked with a higher likelihood of developing cancer, heart disease, and obesity.

At the time of its publication in 2005, The China Study (a partnership between researchers in the U.S., U.K. and China) was touted as "one of the most comprehensive nutritional studies ever undertaken."[5] Researchers surveyed a total 10,200 adults and their families living in rural China and consuming a largely plant-based diet to study the relationship between dietary intake and overall health outcomes for heart disease, diabetes and cancer. Findings of The China Study support recommendations for a plant-based, whole food diet.

One reason this study is so impressive is that it uncovered thousands of significant correlations between dietary intake, other lifestyle factors, and various chronic diseases. We must not forget that "correlation does not equal causation." That is, we cannot say that eating excess amounts of animal-based proteins causes cancer or heart disease. However, excessive intake and an overall unbalanced diet are likely to increase the odds of developing these leading causes of death.

More broadly speaking, another inherent challenge of nutrition research is the difficulty of measuring the synergistic effect of foods and completely controlling for confounding variables.[6] In other words, it is difficult to understand how the combined effects of a varied diet are protective or harmful while adequately controlling all of the other variables that may contribute to confusing or sometimes misleading results. Therefore, we should not use The China Study as a guide to determine what constitutes an optimal diet, rather this monumental study should stand as a testament to temperance. The importance of having a balanced and varied diet cannot be overstated and this is the lesson one should take from The China Study.

We know that regularly eating excessive amounts of protein is not a good approach for the long-term health of the kidneys. Let's not forget just how important this organ is for the body to naturally detoxify and promote overall health. When one regularly eats high intakes of protein — far in excess of estimated needs — this requires the kidneys to work harder to process the proteins and rid the body of nitrogenous waste (a byproduct of protein digestion). This is particularly true for those who have chronic kidney disease. On the contrary, in various smaller-scale randomized controlled trials, researchers found that a high-protein, low carbohydrate diet can help with weight loss and may even improve blood pressure or elevated triglycerides.[7] However, these positive effects were modest and researchers did not consider potential long-term adverse effects of the diet on health and longevity.

Despite the ongoing debate about what is an optimal balance of macronutrients (carbohydrates, proteins, and dietary fats), there is limited evidence that suggests higher intakes of animal-based proteins is significantly correlated with mortality (increased chances of dying earlier) in people between ages 50–65. Whereas, higher protein intake in those 65 years and older may have some protective effects and reduce the chances of cancer and mortality.[8] These contrasting findings suggest that lower protein intake in middle age may be protective, while lower or inadequate intakes in elderly people (>65 years old) may have more harmful effects on health and longevity. Although these results may seem confusing to some, again the lesson here is about the importance of eating a balanced diet and not eating *too much of a good thing*.

Another point: it's very common for people to overestimate their protein needs and eat much more than needed. It's common for personal trainers to recommend one to two grams of protein per pound of body weight. This recommendation far exceeds what a scientific consensus suggests is adequate protein for most people. If you are not a strength or endurance athlete, training for a marathon, or have some sort of hypermetabolic condition occurring, then about 0.8 – 1 gram of protein per *kilogram* of body weight is estimated as adequate to support health and muscle development. For example, a healthy adult female weighing 140 pounds (about 64 kilograms), needs approximately 50-65 grams of protein per day (64 x 0.8 to 64 x 1.0). This is far less than the 140 to 280 grams some fitness professionals might erroneously recommend to this 140-pound woman. This excessive — and unrealistic for some — amount of protein intake will displace other varied, nutrient-dense foods we *should* be eating for optimal health.

In summary, consuming adequate protein intake is very important throughout life; however, regularly eating amounts in excess of estimated needs is likely to have more harmful, than helpful, consequences in the long-run.

Besides excessive protein intake, a similar concern can be said about eating too much of other healthy foods, such as fruits, starchy vegetables, or whole grains. This is especially true when these foods are processed into low-fiber food products, such as juices, potato chips or crackers. A diet consisting primarily of high carb foods (including higher sugar fruits, starchy vegetables and refined grains) and suboptimal amounts of protein, fiber, and fats can contribute to metabolic disturbances. Specifically, this unbalanced food intake can promote weight gain and problems with blood sugar regulation, eventually promoting obesity and even pre-diabetes or diabetes. Likewise, by drinking a lot of juices instead of regularly eating whole fruits, the higher concentration of sugar intake can also promote metabolic disturbances, in other words, a disruption of a normal blood sugar balance. Sure, you might still get some important vitamins and minerals from drinking some juices, though the lack of fiber and a higher concentration of natural sugars (or added sugars) is what can contribute to irregular blood sugar levels and weight gain.

PRINCIPLE 3:
KEEP IT SIMPLE - PLANTS ARE GOOD

Let's move past some of the confusing or unsettled research about protein intake and acknowledge one underlying tenet most researchers can agree on. With few exceptions, whole foods, mostly plant-based and in their unprocessed (or minimally processed) state are good for you and essential for good health. Considering a balanced dietary pattern that can improve overall health and mental well-being, one common ground among a variety of different healthy eating patterns is a greater reliance on a variety of fruits, vegetables, and other high-fiber plant-based food staples.

Although there are no particular fruits or vegetables that you must eat, it's important to have a good variety, especially including different colors as often as possible. In general, the darker the color of the plant-based, whole food the more nutrient-dense it is. For example, dark leafy greens such as spinach, kale, or broccoli tend to be some of the veggies with the highest amount of nutrients (vitamins and minerals). Similarly, berries tend to be some of the most nutrient-dense fruits available. However, don't just focus on these select few, eat a variety of fruits and vegetables as often as you can!

Or, if you have certain gastrointestinal disorders, these high-fiber foods should be eaten as often as tolerated as you may need to include more of these plant-based whole-foods at a more strategic and cautionary rate, perhaps even avoiding certain ones for certain periods of time. Again, one must not forget about the importance of addressing and treating any underlying gastrointestinal issues before adding too many high-fiber plant-based foods to the diet. Even for those without more significant gastrointestinal issues, sometimes making dramatic dietary changes too fast can result in abdominal discomfort or worse symptoms in some other situations. This is particularly true for those who don't drink enough water or other unsweetened, non-caffeinated beverages and add too much fiber too quickly. So make sure to first drink plenty of water before you add too much fiber to your diet.

You might think I'm advocating a vegan or vegetarian diet here. Let me be clear that I am not, despite that many (certainly not all) food and nutrition experts might argue that either a strictly or mostly-plant-based diet (i.e. veganism or various forms of vegetarianism) is the best way to optimize health through dietary changes. For some, this might be the best dietary approach. For others, it might not be. However, the important point again is that I am not attempting to determine any sort of perfect diet for health. Rather, this chapter is about cutting through the confusion and focusing more on the common ground about what constitutes a healthy diet that contributes to improved mental well-being in conjunction with other lifestyle changes on your journey. In the spirit of balance and temperance, you might consider this idea of an optimal diet as the "flexitarian" diet, which mostly emphasizes whole foods, plant-based.

Besides the exclusive criteria of what one might think of when they imagine a vegan or vegetarian diet, another way to consider this more inclusive healthy dietary pattern is a "plant-forward" way of eating. This term was coined through a public health initiative from one of the leaders in academia in partnership with one of the most prestigious culinary schools in America. The Department of Nutrition at Harvard T.H. Chan School of Public Health paired up with the Culinary Institute of America to develop "plant-forward" eating.[9] Or, as put even more simply by the renowned journalist, author and activist Michael Pollan, "Eat food. Not too much. Mostly plants."[10]

CHAPTER 7

CRAFTING YOUR FOODS FOR THOUGHT GAME PLAN

Simply put, the diet or eating pattern that works for you is the one for you. There's no one best diet that will work for all people. Nor is there a single diet that is compliant with a wide variety of dietary restrictions or religious or cultural preferences. Dietary needs and preferences are influenced by a variety of factors, such as pre-existing digestive problems, genetic and cultural backgrounds, just to name a few. Therefore, the best dietary advice to one person may be unhelpful advice to another.

The dietary pattern that's most appealing and best for you might be different from what your friend follows, swears by, and attributes all their health progress and success to. Everybody has their own unique preferences, abilities, and motivations for making healthy lifestyle changes. Find a healthy dietary pattern or model that not only sounds appealing to you but one that will also work with your lifestyle. One that takes into consideration your individual strengths and skills as well as your own unique challenges and barriers that sometimes prevent you from following a healthy plan.

Furthermore, and to reiterate, mental well-being and attaining optimal treatment outcomes is not all about just eating a healthy diet. If it were this simple, mental health would not be the magnitude of the problem that it is around the world today. The first part of crafting your *Foods for Thought Game Plan* is to take stock of your health and well-being (see *dimensions of wellness* in Afterword). Once you have identified what practices of self-care and other areas of wellness you can improve on, set a more specific plan of how you will improve these other interconnected aspects of your health that need the most work. Some keys to accomplishing this — along with dietary changes — include knowing your limitations and what motivates you, setting SMART goals (discussed below), establishing a solid social support system, and utilizing any resources as necessary to help you overcome barriers and accomplish your goals. Over time, as you build more confidence and success from accomplishing these smaller goals, these baby steps turn into significant, lasting, and life-changing improvements in health and overall quality of life. Not only do such lifestyle changes improve *your* health but they can also greatly benefit the health and quality of life of your loved ones as well.

BEFORE CHANGES, KNOW YOUR LIMITATIONS

As you craft your *Foods for Thought Game Plan*, there are several things to consider that could pose barriers if not addressed first. Clarifying the obstacles that stand in your way can help you determine your best approach towards lifestyle changes. Consider each of the following five factors listed below to determine which areas are in most need of improvement. With this information, you can then find more assistance or resources to promote success along your health journey.

1. ***Budget restraints*** Can you afford to purchase all the food you would like on a regular basis? Do you need to sometimes borrow money to feed the family, or do you use resources to stretch the food budget, such as community-supported agriculture systems (CSAs), Supplemental Nutrition and Assistance Program (SNAP, a federal program, previously referred to as "food stamps"), or other similar local or state food assistance? If food

insecurity is an obstacle to healthy changes, you may need to look into community resources and see what is available in your region. For example, in Arizona where I grew up, throughout most of the year, a collective group of farmers donates or sells their produce at a low cost. Though this local cooperative does cost about $12 each trip, consumers walk away with a haul of seventy pounds of produce, great value for those who take the time to prepare, store, and utilize all this healthy produce.

2. ***Time restraints*** On an average week, how much time do you usually spend grocery shopping, preparing food, and cleaning up? Do you often not have enough time to eat healthfully, yet spend two to four hours on an average day scrolling through your social media feeds, playing video games, watching television, or online videos? Sometimes time restraints are more a matter of not choosing daily activities that align well with what a person's stated personal values or goals are. If time is a barrier to your healthy changes, maybe it's a good idea to take inventory of where you spend most of your leisure time and find some extra time to shop, prepare, and cook healthy meals. This is a process. Try and be patient and understand that lifestyle changes aren't always as fast and efficient as we would like them to be.

3. ***Cooking skills/kitchen access*** In modern American culture, unfortunately, many people grow up without learning basic cooking and kitchen skills. Therefore, it's common to feel lost following recipes or preparing whole foods from scratch at home. If this is your biggest barrier to making healthy changes, maybe start more gradually or start with simple changes, such as committing to prepare one to three new meals per week by following recipes you've never tried. If you don't like eating fruits or vegetables, consider making smoothies for an easy and convenient way to get more of these nutrient-dense food staples.

4. ***Support system*** Do you have others that you can count on for their support in challenging times, to hold you accountable and motivate you to stick with healthy changes rather than dissuade you or perhaps even encourage old unhealthy habits? If not, there's plenty of people out there in similar situations who would be happy to pair up with you. Whether virtually with online support or even finding a Meetup group online to join in person. Find people with common goals and lifestyles that you would like to meet and make new friends.

5. ***Commitment level*** How committed are you to your lifestyle changes? Are you brand new to changing your diet and practicing lifestyle changes? Have you been trying to diet for years? What really motivates you to make these healthy changes? These can be tough questions to answer. However, if your level of commitment is the biggest area for improvement, then perhaps you are not ready to invest your time and energy in significant lifestyle changes, and this is okay. Everybody makes changes at their own pace! Sometimes, exploring the reasons why you want to change a behavior in the first place is a good point to start to understand what motivates you. Or maybe sticking with more basic SMART goals is a better approach if you just don't feel as committed as you would like at this time. It is better to commit to smaller goals and accomplish them over time rather than setting overly ambitious, unrealistic goals that often lead to feelings of failure or disappointment.

KNOW WHAT MOTIVATES YOU

Are you making these dietary changes simply because your doctor told you to but not really sure why else you should stick with these changes? Or perhaps you recently came to the realization that what you've eaten and your lifestyle over the past several years (or decades) is likely the biggest contributor to some of your most serious health concerns and you are ready to make whatever change is necessary to feel better. Your concerns may be about digestive health, overall physical health, or even depression or anxiety, without much other explanation as to the underlying causes of these mental health disorders. Everybody has their unique concerns about health, understanding of the effectiveness of health changes, and perceptions of the severity of health problems and importance of lifestyle changes. What is highly motivating to one person might not begin to motivate another person. If you're not already clear on what exactly motivates you, spend some time thinking about this. Write it down. When we don't remind ourselves about the "why" behind making such lifestyle changes, these changes can seem more challenging or even annoying, even sometimes rising to the level of resentment and resulting in negative self-talk such as "it's just not worth it", or "I'll just eat whatever I want anyhow."

SETTING SMART GOALS

SMART goals are Specific, Measurable, Attainable, Realistic, and Time-bound.[1] It's important to set SMART goals because if you set a non-specific goal, such as "I will eat more vegetables", how can you hold yourself accountable to whether or not you really accomplished it? Setting SMART goals can help you accomplish overall health goals in a timely, effective manner. Think of these goals as steps along your journey. This builds confidence in the process and helps you become more aware of your successes and the benefits you experience from your hard work invested.

For some, small steps might mean first reducing your soda intake and increasing your water intake for a month before you commit to changing the foods you eat. Over time, success from these "baby steps" helps you realize a clearer vision of other goals you would like to achieve. Keep in mind that setting and accomplishing SMART goals is an ongoing process. Be flexible with this process and learn to adopt different goals that are more fitting to your lifestyle. When you accomplish one or two SMART goals, move on to the next whenever you feel ready to do so.

The SMART goals you set should not only focus on healthy dietary changes, but they might also include goals to begin a regular practice of stretching in the mornings or a ten-minute walk after dinner at least four or five days per week, or whatever type of physical activity is more than what you're currently doing. Set some sort of physical fitness goal and get to work. You are physically capable of so much more than you realize, it just takes time and discipline to gradually realize your potential. So take time to explore what you are truly capable of by beginning exercise and fitness "low and slow." That is, practice a low-intensity activity for a short duration of time, but do it more frequently if you want better results. You can think of accomplishing these SMART goals as baby steps towards a healthier lifestyle and improved mental well-being.

SMART goals

- Specific - detail specifically what you would like to accomplish
- Measurable - the ability to measure your stated goal and outcomes
- Attainable - is the goal attainable considering your unique barriers, limitations, etc.?
- Realistic - is the goal realistic given your current resources, availability, commitment?
- Time-bound - a set amount of time or duration is included to accomplish the goal

---

To illustrate this, one example of a generic (non-SMART) goal is "*I will eat less fried foods.*" How can one really understand what this means? How can you measure whether or not this was accomplished?

Sure, this might be *Attainable* and *Realistic* but it's also not a *Time-bound* goal, so when do we ask whether or not the goal was accomplished? A more practical example of a SMART goal might be *"I will limit the soda to less than or equal to two cans per week for the next month."* This latter goal is more likely to result in successful changes.

OR, "CLEAN HOUSE AND DIVE IN"

On the other hand, maybe you're feeling really confident about investing in lifestyle changes, have a strong support system, and don't have any major barriers or health conditions to first remedy. Or perhaps you've already made great changes in the past and know exactly what it takes and just need to "get back on track." You might feel ready to dive in or follow a specific meal plan more rigidly with discipline and structure. This type of approach might include emptying out your refrigerator and cabinets of any "junk foods." For some people, this rigid adherence to healthy diet and exercise plans may result in frustration and lack of long-term results from not sticking with it. For others, following a structured plan is the most effective and life-changing approach and just the thing they need to maintain success and adherence to set plans.

Whatever you determine your best approach is, remember, this is not about perfecting your diet. Over time you can modify what is working well and what is not working so well. Keep this in mind in case your strict adherence to any diet plan ever begins to trigger self-critical thoughts and your sense of "falling off track" results in critical thoughts such as "forget it, I'll just eat whatever I want anyhow."

DIETARY MODELS

Note that I use the word *models* here rather than just *diets*. This is because having a healthy relationship with food and eating healthfully should not require a person to eat only certain foods or entire food groups and completely avoid others. There are exceptions for people with allergies who need to avoid certain foods, or those following elimination trials, such as for determining suspected food intolerances, ruling out allergies, etc. However, as stated several times earlier in this book, it's the pattern that is more important, and so we'll look at a few different model dietary patterns — dietary models that have been proven effective at helping to improve measures of heart disease, diabetes, obesity, and other chronic inflammatory diseases. As you know by now, what is good for controlling chronic inflammation, in turn, is likely helpful for improving symptoms of depression.

DASH Diet

Originally established to target reduction of blood pressure, DASH (Dietary Approaches to Stop Hypertension) is a balanced eating plan that limits sodium, allows flexibility, and does not require you to eat particular foods.[2] Rather, this plan specifies how many servings you need daily of each food group (based on your estimated daily calorie needs), what constitutes a serving, and what are healthy choices for each of the recommended food groups. This diet is thought to be helpful for treating hypertension and good for heart health, not only due to controlled intakes of sodium and saturated fats, but also from the adequate intake and variety of fruits, vegetables, whole grains, legumes, and nuts or seeds. These various nutrient-dense plant-based foods help provide the body with greater amounts of dietary fiber and key minerals like potassium and magnesium, which are all linked to blood pressure and heart health.

It's not just the heart and overall cardiovascular system that this eating plan is beneficial for. Now recommended by the Alzheimer's Association, DASH is considered a healthy dietary plan for brain health and helping to delay or prevent neurodegenerative diseases such as Alzheimer's disease. Although the relationship between cognitive function and diet is not very clear in research, it is not a far stretch to think what is good for the overall health of the heart and brain, is also helpful for general mental well-being. If you're interested in following the DASH diet, there's a lot of great resources available online (check out Resources at the end of the book) that specify your individual needs for each food group, per caloric needs, and instruct you on how to craft a meal plan.

Mediterranean Diet

Despite the word "diet" here, the Mediterranean diet is not a diet per se, rather it's a healthy dietary pattern commonly seen among those who live along the Mediterranean Sea. According to the *U.S. News & World Report*, the Mediterranean diet was the "Best Overall for Healthy Eating" and the "Easiest to Follow" among other healthy diets reviewed for 2018, 2019, and 2020.[3] Remember the healthy populations of the Blue Zones discussed in Chapter 6? Sardinia, one of the Blue Zones, is an Italian island located in the Mediterranean Sea. Similar to the DASH diet, the Mediterranean diet is considered healthy mostly thanks to the abundance of nutrient-dense whole foods included in their minimally processed forms. This "diet" emphasizes eating a variety of fruits, vegetables, whole grains, legumes, nuts, olive oil, and, of course, flavorful herbs and spices to bring the dishes to life. This greatly contrasts with the "standard American diet" by avoiding too much high-fat meat and too many dairy and highly processed food products that are packed with harmful processed oils and refined grains that don't nourish or satisfy us as much. Note that the Mediterranean diet is loaded with plenty of foods and essential fats that not only nourish your brain, but they also nourish your second brain by providing the various sources of indigestible fiber that our friendly gut bugs need to keep doing their job and contributing to our health.

Anti-Inflammatory Diet

After discussing the DASH and Mediterranean diet, the lines start to get blurry between these diets and the "anti-inflammatory diet."[4] In other words, there are many more similarities between each of these rather than differences. Like the previous two dietary patterns, the anti-inflammatory diet emphasizes a good variety of nutrient-dense fruits and vegetables that have been shown to demonstrate anti-inflammatory effects, especially emphasizing dark leafy greens, berries, and yellow/red/orange vegetables. The anti-inflammatory diet instructs us to avoid foods that can contribute to chronic inflammation. This makes it different from the other two because it limits or avoids gluten-containing or refined grains and other pro-inflammatory foods, including highly processed food products loaded with refined oils and refined grains. This diet also limits red meat and dairy products that are high in saturated fats and may contribute to inflammation.

Now, the common theme should start to become clear about what constitutes a healthy and balanced diet that is good for overall health, and good for the health of the brain and the gut.

MIND Diet Project

Short of establishing dietary guidelines for mental health, researchers are in the process of conducting interventional and clinical trials and, therefore, further establishing evidence to outline what we might someday use as prescribed diets for brain health and treatment of mental health disorders.

Researchers at Rush University in Chicago and Harvard T.H. Chan School of Public Health teamed-up to study the effects of diet on Alzheimer's disease and cognitive decline associated with aging.[5] The MIND diet (Mediterranean-DASH Intervention for Neurodegenerative Delay) developed by this group defines how many servings of each food group should be eaten daily or weekly. It combines the Mediterranean and DASH eating patterns we have previously covered.

One study published by these researchers investigated the diet–Alzheimer's disease link in a group of 923 subjects assigned to three different diets (MIND, Mediterranean and DASH) over an average

4.5 years. Analyzing the data from this observational study, researchers concluded, closely following any of these three diets — MIND, Mediterranean, or DASH — may reduce risk of Alzheimer's disease. [6]

In another MIND-diet study, the researchers examined cognitive decline among participants in the Memory and Aging Project. Results suggested that the MIND diet "substantially slows cognitive decline with age."[7] We need additional studies of this type — longer-term and with a greater number of participants — yielding similar results before we can say with confidence that the MIND diet is the one most likely to slow age-related cognitive decline.

Although more research is needed to confirm the findings of both studies, the MIND diet stands as a potential model diet we might use to protect brain health. In turn, it's not a far stretch to think this diet may hold potential for improving mental health outcomes.

SMILES Trial

Moving beyond observational research and looking towards the future, the SMILES trial (Supporting the Modification of Lifestyle in Lowered Emotional States) was a first-of-its-kind randomized controlled trial that aimed to study the effects of structured dietary changes, along with nutrition consultations with a clinical dietitian, in those with moderate to severe depression. Despite some limitations, this small study, conducted in Australia and published in 2017, found statistically significant improvements in depressive symptoms in those in the dietary intervention group.[8]

Although the science behind the food-mood connection has only become clearer in recent years, the improvements for symptoms of depression or anxiety that one can feel after diet changes can happen fast, and can be quite impactful. In my experience as a clinical dietitian, countless people have expressed how much better they feel after just a few weeks of changing their daily food choices. In the past few years, I've worked primarily, one-on-one, with people who deal with anxiety and/or depression. Through my personal work of supporting the lifestyle modification — by way of fitness, diet, and connecting people to behavioral health professionals or socioeconomic resources as needed — results can be life-chasnging! Whether it's "I feel so much better", "I'm sleeping through the night", or "I can get up to play with the kids now", some of the benefits to mental well-being from eating a well-balanced diet are difficult to measure in a scientific study.

CONCLUSION

In case you haven't noticed a common theme by now, there are not many easy answers throughout this book. But the message is simple enough: Identify your biggest areas for improvement, target them, and develop a strategy and a game plan for successful results. The few chosen dietary patterns discussed in this chapter are only a few of the examples of healthy dietary models you might choose to navigate through your lifestyle changes and journey towards improved mental well-being.

This final chapter reviewed a few dietary models that have recently shown potential to improve mood and symptoms of depression, and could later serve as effective dietary models to reduce, or even prevent, depression. The potential benefits of these model diets are much greater if you first take the time to read about, and apply, the self-care strategies I describe in the Afterword.

At the end of the book you will find the Resources section to help jumpstart your journey. Consider these resources as a toolbox for planning and practicing your *Foods for Thought Game Plan* and overcoming any obstacles you may experience along the way. Use the right tools you need to accomplish your goals. From recipes to meal plans to inspirational stories, more in-depth instructions about whichever dietary pattern you choose to follow, and much more. These tools can help you find the right resources and can even help you develop a support system on your wellness journey, all the while building confidence, adopting lifestyle changes, and ultimately, achieving better results towards your desired health outcomes. Remember that making sustainable lifestyle changes *is not about* following a rigid plan, eating a "perfect diet", or vowing never again to eat another bag of chips, slice of pizza, or candy bar.

This book is about identifying significant pieces of the puzzle in your journey towards improved health and mental well-being. By this point in the book, I hope you have learned some of the pieces in your puzzle. In other words, I hope you're becoming clear about your personal areas for improvement and realizing how you can invest in lifestyle changes. Through discovering these lifestyle and behavior links, you are now given an opportunity to make important changes. These gradual changes you invest in and accomplish can also influence the lifestyles and health of your loved ones and result in big picture changes that may further improve the quality of life and mental well-being.

Whether it's whole foods plant-based or the Pegan Diet or the GAPS Diet, the Nordic Diet, or whatever else is being talked about by the time you're reading this, these are dietary models or theories that hold various degrees of potential for contributing to optimal health, and may even hold potential for healing the gut from complex life-altering gastrointestinal conditions. However, rather than focusing on the shortcomings of these diets or getting lost in disagreements about how each of these might be "wrong", moving forward let's focus more on the common ground amongst all the prevailing dietary models and theories purported by some of the leading thinkers and practitioners in these areas of research. Finding what works for you and what doesn't work is a personal matter. Hence, no easy answers here. But one of the most promising lessons to take home from this journey in improving your health and mental well-being is that change and progress are possible and within reach regardless of where you're at in your journey today.

Remember that lifestyle changes are an ongoing process and you are stronger than you give yourself credit for! The hard part is just learning what this really means to you and determining your path. Be kind to yourself and be humble. All of the greatest journeys, discoveries, and inventions in history had one thing in common: The exact path forward was unknown. Every pioneer, leader, or discoverer started their journey one step at a time. So don't be intimidated, however grand or minimal you might consider your journey. Develop your *Foods for Thought Game Plan* and take that first step. Learn to re-strategize over time and keep stepping forward, regardless of what stands in your way.

AFTERWORD

SELF-CARE & WELLNESS
(ALL THAT OTHER IMPORTANT HEALTH STUFF)

By reading this book, I hope you have learned that making healthy changes is a highly individualized process (or at least it should be!). There's no perfect diet or best formula to follow for making healthy lifestyle changes that works for everybody. I have identified some of the most common lifestyle factors that contribute to poor overall health. I will discuss the importance of these factors in relation to a holistic, or "whole-person", model of overall health, which can impact mental health. In this book I have shown that what is harmful to your physical well-being is also harmful to other aspects of your overall wellness and, therefore, may negatively impact your emotional wellness and overall mental health.

I have explored aspects of health and wellness that contribute to mental health and should be addressed before making any significant diet changes. If you want to improve your diet and your mental health, it's necessary to take note of areas that need improvement in your overall state of well-being.

SELF-CARE

What comes to your mind when you read the words "self-care"? This term can mean quite a variety of things to different people. Self-care includes routine preventive care: daily practices of brushing and flossing your teeth, stretching, meditating, running, walking the dog, and, of course, eating a healthy diet. For some, self-care might mean following a plan to quit smoking cigarettes and finding healthier habits like walking or practicing yoga instead. For others, this might mean taking their diabetes medications and insulin as prescribed. Or starting to eat breakfast on a regular basis, walking for 15 minutes after dinner, or simply making sure to drink plenty of water every day. Although there is no right or wrong, or best approach or formula to follow that works for everybody, the point here is that regular practice of self-care (whatever this means to you) is important to physical and emotional health; therefore, it's foundational to promoting good mental health.

Some of the most basic, universal means of self-care are adequate rest, physical activity, protecting the brain by avoiding head injuries and substance abuse, stress management, and practicing mindfulness techniques. Lastly, I'll discuss "wellness" (which may overlap with self-care). We'll take a closer look at each of these self-care factors and the "Eight Dimensions of Wellness."[1]

Adequate Rest: Recharge Your Battery

Getting adequate sleep and allowing the body to rest, especially after a stressful day, is essential to promote a healthy body and a healthy mind. You should not overlook this basic act of self-care when taking charge of your health and learning to improve current mental health through lifestyle changes. You may not notice the effects of getting poor sleep if this is your norm, but it can have both short-term and long-term effects on your health. Besides the more immediate effects of fatigue, poor mood, or difficulty with concentrating, a chronic lack of sleep is associated with high blood pressure, diabetes, and heart disease. These are just a few of the greatest causes of death for most Americans.[2] Although we can't say that a lack of sleep directly causes these chronic diseases, the correlations are important because they help us understand how harmful chronic poor sleep may be on long-term physical health.

During sleep, the body repairs and rebuilds from different types of stress that you encounter throughout the day, both physical and mental. In other words, sleep is restorative and allows the cells of the body to reset natural hormonal regulation and restore any damage that normally happens on a daily basis. Keep this in mind when increasing your exercise regimen because exercise is stressful to the body, and the more physical activity you do the more important that restful sleep is. Therefore, it's not only the exercise itself, but adequate sleep and refueling of your body (and brain) with nutrient-dense foods after exercise that allows the body to overcome stress and get stronger, and ultimately achieve the results and goals you've set and worked hard for. Similar to a rechargeable battery, if you don't recharge (restful sleep) your battery (mind and body), you either cannot perform your daily tasks as effectively as you would like to, or your best intentions to accomplish those tasks will fall short.

Unfortunately, many people suffer from insomnia or other sleep disorders. This can make the simple advice of getting adequate sleep on most nights very difficult to accomplish. In fact, nearly one out of every five Americans has either a sleep disorder or wakefulness disorder (e.g. narcolepsy, obstructive sleep apnea, restless leg syndrome, and insomnia).[3] Compared to "normal sleepers," a 2014 study showed that older adults with chronic insomnia were between four to ten times more likely to experience depression when interviewed at follow-up surveys.[4] For those who suffer from sleep and wakefulness disorders, working with a medical doctor is an important first step in addressing such disorders. However, people often don't realize (or doctors might not advise the patient) how much of their daily habits and nightly routines can sabotage the body's natural sleep cycle and disrupt the quality and pattern of sleep. In other words, they may have poor sleep hygiene habits. By modifying a few behaviors and daily routines, improvements in quality and duration of sleep often will follow.

The National Institutes for Health recommends at least 7-8 hours of sleep per night for most adults. Complete a sleep diary to help reflect on your sleep hygiene and identify ways to help improve your quality of sleep (found at sleepeducation.org).[5] By completing this two-week diary, you can find insight to help identify how your lifestyle impacts your ability to attain adequate, restful sleep. Also, consider the following tips to help you establish a relaxing bedtime routine.[6]

Sleep Hygiene Tips:

- Make your bedroom a relaxing, comfortable setting with a cool temperature
- Maintain a consistent sleep schedule (same bedtime, wake time every day)
- Beds are for sleep (and sex) only, not for watching TV before sleep time
- Limit exposure to bright lights at least two hours before bedtime
- Avoid screen time (phone, computer, TV, etc.) at least 1–2 hours before bedtime
- Avoid caffeine in late afternoon and evening
- Exercise regularly (adequate physical stress helps induce restful sleep)
- Avoid consuming alcohol and reduce water intake before bed
- Avoid eating large meals within a couple of hours before bedtime
- Aromatherapy for relaxation (using essential oils)
  - o   Lavender
  - o   Jasmine, bergamot, and ylang ylang are sometimes used[7]

Although you might feel fine after little sleep (especially if you are young), the true cost to your health from chronic poor sleep is difficult to fully understand and should not be overlooked. The optimal amount of sleep can feel different from person to person, particularly varying between different stages of life (e.g. infants, developing children, and growing teenagers need more sleep than middle-aged adults) and your activity level. However, about seven to nine hours of quality sleep per night is adequate for most adults.[8] So make sure to plan a sleeping schedule and relaxing nighttime routine that allows you at least seven hours of quality sleep per night.

Physical Activity/Exercise

Exercise and physical activity may be the cheapest and most under-rated, all-natural form of antidepressant and anti-anxiety remedy readily available! Epidemiological research (conducted on large populations that identify correlations between different behaviors; does not establish cause and effect) suggests that physical activity is the most commonly identified behavior that has a positive impact on sleep.[9] As we just noted, the importance of restful sleep for promoting mental wellbeing cannot be overstated. Therefore, physical activity not only has a more direct impact on mood (discussed later) but also can have an indirect impact on mental health by improving sleep quality.

Some of the proposed mechanisms by which exercise promotes a positive mental state are increasing blood flow and delivery of oxygen to the brain, and increasing the body's ability to tolerate stress. Improved tolerance to stress helps you better deal with and overcome everyday stressors. It helps you not to perceive everyday stressors as harmful or threatening, as you might usually do, whether you realize it or not.

Regarding the stress response, the Hypothalamic-Pituitary-Adrenal (HPA)-axis is the primary biological system involved in the body's perception of and response to stress. This term describes different areas in the brain (hypothalamus, pituitary gland) that "communicate" with the adrenal glands, the hormonal system of the kidneys. This link is important because these specific regions in the brain involved with communication and coordination of the HPA-axis are also known to control mood and motivation and influence fear related to stress and anxiety.[10] To simplify a confusing concept: practicing consistent and frequent exercise — along with adequate rest and refueling with nutritious foods — helps the HPA-axis stay within its normal range of functioning and thus promotes a sense of emotional well-being. This can translate to improved chronic stress management and decreased symptoms of anxiety or depression.

The benefits of regular exercise to mental health may be derived from a variety of other factors. In addition to improved flow of oxygen and enhanced stress response, exercise can increase mental well-being by improving sleep, sexual desire, stamina, and mental alertness. Throughout my years as a personal trainer, the fastest achieved and most common benefit I would usually hear clients report after beginning an exercise regimen was improved sleep! Furthermore, exercise helps to maintain a healthy weight or assist with weight loss, which can also serve to increase self-esteem and confidence to set more advanced goals with physical activities. These benefits of exercise can prove helpful for different mood disorders and could be a missing key in your lifestyle when you suffer from anxiety and/or depression and do not do any regular physical activity.

For those who are new to fitness and have not exercised much in the past, this is okay. It's important to balance adequate physical activities (including non-exercise activities) with inactivity and rest. This means don't do too much too quickly when it comes to starting a new exercise regimen. Now knowing the importance of adequate rest (discussed above), it's especially important for beginners and those who haven't regularly exercised for many years, to begin low and slow with exercise. In other words, begin with something low intensity and for a short duration of time.

If you haven't walked more than two blocks at once in two years, it's probably not a good idea to go and try to run two miles. A better and more effective approach is to set a goal to walk for ten to thirty minutes at least four times per week, and do it! Then, after two to three weeks of practicing this, you will have built confidence and endurance and after this point (and with the release from your physician) you can set and accomplish greater goals. You are capable of so much more than you give yourself credit for. But be patient and make a consistent and solid effort with exercise and you will get stronger and eventually see results.

Some basics to think about when determining a good regimen is *the F.I.T.T. formula:* Frequency, Intensity, Timing and Type.

Frequency

How many times per week can you realistically commit to exercise? Exercising seven days a week is probably too much and is overtraining for most people. On the other hand, one to two times per week may not be enough. Your optimal frequency (i.e., how often you exercise per week) may change from time to time depending on your goals, barriers, time restraints, etc.

Intensity

How intense or difficult is the activity? For example, for most people cardio exercise should be lower intensity, and you should be able to maintain a moderate conversation during activity. Resistance training should be higher intensity, done with good form and slow, controlled movements. Typically, heart rate is measured during exercise to determine intensity.

Timing

How long is your session, or each component of exercise? For example, when working on stretching (flexibility training) after workouts, aim for holding each stretch between thirty to sixty seconds. In order to get more benefit from cardio, exercise should be of moderate intensity, yet prolonged for at least fifteen to twenty minutes (except for those who are brand new to exercise or have other certain medical conditions not cleared by doctor) in order to get conditioned to lower levels of physical activity first.

Type

What type of activity do you like to do? If you want to improve your cardiovascular (aerobic) ability, maybe swimming, biking, running, or jogging is the best type of exercise to focus more on. If you want to lose weight, maybe you need a combination of resistance training, flexibility, and cardio exercises.

Protecting Your Brain

Improving your mental wellbeing is not only about eating a balanced, nutrient-dense diet that provides the brain with the key building blocks it requires to feel well; it's also about protecting the brain from overexposure to things that can cause harm. Oxidants are byproducts naturally produced in the body. When too many oxidants or too much oxidative stress build up and are not regulated it can cause damage to DNA and proteins. Damage to DNA and proteins in the body is one thing that can cause disease and illness. Too much exposure to certain foods (particularly deep-fried foods), heavy metals, and other environmental pollutants can increase the amount of oxidative stress to the cells of the body and the brain. Left unchecked, over time, oxidative damage in the brain can increase the likelihood of developing Alzheimer's disease. Most people are exposed on a daily basis to factors, such as excessive stress, toxins, and potentially harmful chemicals in various self-care products that cause oxidative stress. Without a healthy diet, the body has less capacity to effectively deal with this stress load. Many of the vitamins, minerals, antioxidants, and phytonutrients in foods have important protective effects for your brain and can help to combat exposure to these brain pollutants. This points to one of the themes of this book, which is the importance of a balanced diet that includes a variety of nutrient-dense fruits, vegetables, and other plant-based whole foods.

Beyond the preventive approach of a healthy diet, there is more you can do to protect your brain. Avoid smoking cigarettes as this is one of the biggest ways of exposing the body and brain to an onslaught of oxidants, heavy metals, and other toxic chemicals. Some other "brain agers" that can cause harm to the brain cells are also considered oxidants, such as excess alcohol and chronic stress. Remember that oxidants are a natural byproduct of stress or exposure to environmental pollutants and toxins. When the body lacks an adequate supply of antioxidants from healthy foods and is overcome by too many oxidants, this can eventually pose problems for brain health.[11]

Stress—Manage It or It Manages You

Too much stress can be a killer. However, some stress is normal and everybody experiences stress from time to time to various degrees. Simply put, "stress is how the brain and body respond to any demand."[12] With the busy lives of most adults, continually changing from one task to another can result in a general feeling of mental overload. Not managing your stress can promote chronically elevated levels of stress hormones that over time can affect your memory or potentially even increase the chances of getting Alzheimer's disease.[13] Although stress may affect everybody, people cope with stress in various ways; some in more productive and health-promoting ways than others. Examples include finding new healthy habits like establishing an exercise regimen, seeking out a new group of social support/friends with similar health-conscious intentions, or following a healthy dietary pattern (or other self-care measures discussed later in the chapter).

Yoga, meditation, or Tai Chi (discipline of Chinese martial arts) are some effective tools you can learn that have powerful destressing effects. There is no right or wrong way to de-stress. Find what you enjoy, what works for you, and move forward in practice once you find something that fits your lifestyle and desired goals. This gives way to our final example of basic self-care: practicing mindfulness. This is a perfect place to transition to the importance of being more mindful, given that practicing mindfulness is considered among the most effective ways of managing stress.

Practicing Mindfulness

There are many different ways to practice being more mindful. Mindfulness is a term to describe the act of slowing down and intentionally allowing the body and mind to better align. In other words, it's the "practice of purposefully focusing your attention on the present moment — and accepting it without judgment."[14] What comes to your mind when you hear the word meditation? Many people tend to think something along the lines of "I don't know how to meditate." The truth is there are no specific rules you need to follow, but the benefits can be profound to anybody who regularly practices meditation or other similar meditative practices. As little as ten minutes a day or less can make a difference in relaxing the mind and promoting a more restful, calm feeling which can help determine how well you feel the rest of the day.

Whether it's yoga, a walk in the park or other outdoor area, or practicing meditation, there are a variety of different ways to practice mindfulness. This is something that you may never truly appreciate the benefits of until you give it a consistent and solid effort. There is a community of health and nutrition professionals out there who teach the concepts of *mindful eating* or *intuitive eating*. These practices help you slow down while eating. This can help improve digestion and allows time for greater appreciation of the foods you eat while making diet changes. Although this is a relatively new concept in science, nonetheless, researchers are now taking a closer look and examining mindfulness as a potentially effective tool in reducing stress and promoting happiness.

WELLNESS: IT'S NOT JUST DIET AND EXERCISE

In our busy, technology-driven lives today, it's easy to let advertisements and personal news feeds influence emotions and determine where most of our daily attention is spent. A constant, daily bombardment of advertisements and reverence towards the consumption of products and fulfilling consumer needs (however contrived these needs may be) is likely to leave one seeking more superficial values such as more money or purchasing more expensive items to exhibit social status. Or perhaps such purchases might be filling a void we haven't yet fully acknowledged or reconciled. Obtaining some of these more superficial values (e.g. amassing consumer goods) may however pose as a barrier to achieving more fulfilling and impactful goals, or obtaining a greater sense of wellness.

On a deeper level of promoting mental well-being, humans have important psychological needs, such as the need to feel a sense of belonging, to feel valued by other people, and to feel a sense of meaning and purpose in life. Although this subject is beyond the scope of this book, I mention it here to contextualize the importance of daily lifestyle choices. We live in a time of abundance, yet paradoxically depression and anxiety are still major problems that plagues much of the developed world. Hence, wellness can sometimes seem a confusing concept but can actually be pretty basic when it comes to applying daily practices of self-care and contributing bit by bit to your overall sense of well-being.

Now let's move beyond the basic self-care acts previously discussed to a holistic perspective of health and examine the role other lifestyle factors have on mental health and wellness in general. To keep it simple, we can think more broadly of overall health (including physical health, mental health, and beyond) as the concept of *wellness*. Self-care measures are simply behaviors practiced in order to improve one's health; wellness provides the broader picture of overall human health with different aspects (or dimensions) that are interrelated.

The Eight Dimensions of Wellness (Figure 4 below) explains this broader, whole-person model of health.[15] This model recognizes the importance of the following aspects of wellness: 1) emotional, 2) spiritual, 3) intellectual, 4) physical, 5) environmental, 6) financial, 7) occupational, and 8) social. Each of these dimensions of wellness is interrelated and influences the others. In other words, this can be considered a feedback loop because of how influential each component is to the next. For example, if you often worry about making debt payments on time or have overdraft or late fees on a regular basis (financial), this may promote stress and anxiety (emotional). Over time, this anxiety over finances can result in poor sleep quality which may in turn impact your immune system and increase the likelihood of getting sick (physical) or affect the ability to focus at work and hinder performance (occupational).

On the other hand, you can positively impact these interrelated dimensions of wellness, and in turn, improve your mood and your overall health. If you begin a regular exercise routine, this will help

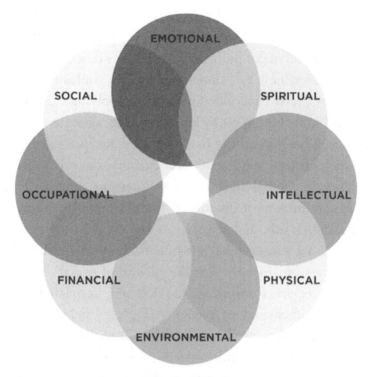

WELLNESS

FIGURE 4. Eight Dimensions of Wellness. This image was adapted by the Substance Abuse and Mental Health Services Administration, U.S. Department of Health and Human Services, from Swarbrick, M. (2006). A Wellness Approach. *Psychiatric Rehabilitation Journal,* 29(4), 311-314.

increase strength and energy and decrease future chances of injuries (physical), which will likely also result in improved sleep quality and improved focus and energy throughout the day (occupational and emotional). Over time, these may help you get more tasks accomplished in the day and this allows for more time to spend on other things you would love to do but do not make enough time for, such as helping with a community garden (environmental, social), reading more books (intellectual), or practicing yoga, meditation, or attending church services more often (spiritual).

As you learn more about this holistic, whole-person model of health, you will gather the knowledge and resources you need to put these principles into practice to improve your health and overall quality of life. Furthermore, as you become more intentional and responsible for your own health outcomes through lifestyle modifications (along with consultation from your primary care provider) you can better manage many different common medical conditions, whether physical health diagnoses or various mental illnesses.

THE EIGHT DIMENSIONS OF WELLNESS
Emotional

The emotional dimension of wellness illustrates the importance of expressing feelings and understanding what your emotional strengths are. Identify aspects of your life in your control that you can modify to boost your emotional well-being. This dimension also speaks to the importance of self-reflection and asking yourself sometimes challenging questions about what and why you do what you do. For example, if you are prioritizing a behavior (such as watching 2-3 hours per night television programs and/or scrolling through the news feed on social media) that limits your best intentions (e.g. your goal to exercise three times per week), over time this may negatively impact your emotional wellness. You might be left with a sense of failure or lack of confidence in your ability to accomplish goals. However, you might think more constructively about your challenging goals, take more responsibility for prioritizing your leisure time, and what tasks you will accomplish first. If you commit to a 20-minute walk prior to beginning your favorite evening television program, posting on social media, or opening your favorite app on the phone; this simple act of prioritizing a healthy behavior (and practicing it) can make other healthy choices easier in the future and build self-confidence as you feel a sense of accomplishment.

The emotional aspect of wellness is so interrelated to the other dimensions that it's best to pause here and reflect on some of your emotional strengths and, perhaps more importantly, on daily activities that may hinder your ability to improve emotional wellness. Note that it's important to practice stress-management techniques and other self-care measures because these are foundational to overall health and can, therefore, help you express and manage emotional concerns.

Emotional wellness self-quiz

When reflecting on your emotional health, answer these three questions:

1. At moments of high stress or anxiety, do you often take time to practice any particular self-care measures? This could be as simple as listening to soothing music, calling a friend, going for a walk, or practicing a breathing exercise or yoga poses. Or whatever else you find relieves stress and is not detrimental to health.

2. Do your relationships with friends and family feel safe enough that you can openly express your feelings without feeling judged at a time that you're feeling really anxious or depressed? If not, this may be an indication that some of your social relationships are more harmful than helpful to your emotional wellness.

3. Do you usually plan or allow yourself time (some, not too much) for things that bring you joy or pleasure? If not, this may indicate you work too much or take wonderful care of loved ones but maybe not good care of yourself and your emotional wellness.

If you answered "no" to more than one of these three questions, this may be an indication there is still some work to be done to improve your sense of emotional wellness.

Physical

How many times a year do you have to visit your primary care doctor? How about your dentist? On average, how many times a year do you get sick and have to miss work? If your answers to these questions are more than you'd like to admit or perhaps too low and you rarely ever see your doctor, maybe this is an indication that you are not taking very good care of your physical wellness. A healthy body facilitates a healthy mind, so we must not overlook the importance of a healthy diet, regular exercise, and practice of other self-care measures discussed later in this chapter. In other words, physical health can promote mental health. This includes regular check-ups with your healthcare provider. But if you're going too often, perhaps this is a sign that you're not doing enough to take better personal responsibility for physical health and just relying too much on providers and medications.

Although different aspects of life can impact physical health, in this book we have mainly considered the critical role that daily food choices and physical activity (to a lesser degree) have on physical health. However, when discussing physical health, we must also acknowledge the importance of adequate sleep, taking medications as prescribed, moderating alcohol and caffeine intake, and avoiding smoking and other substances that may harm physical health.

Intellectual

Perhaps you've heard the old saying "use it or lose it." This saying illustrates the importance of intellectually stimulating your brain. In other words, the brain is similar to a muscle in that it needs a variety of stimulation in order to keep strong and capable of functioning at high capacity (this concept is referred to as neuroplasticity). Likewise, muscles on your body need regular stimulation in order to stay strong and maintain the ability to function at high capacity and prevent injuries.

There are endless ways to intellectually stimulate your brain. Find out what are some of your favorites and put them into practice. Make them a part of your lifestyle, not just something you do for a short period of time. Personal interests vary greatly from person to person. Do some reflection by journaling your thoughts on what you like to learn about, then you might find something joyful to keep your brain active and expand your intellect. Even certain games can be intellectually stimulating to the brain, such as chess or a variety of computer or smartphone apps or similar "brain games."

Perhaps there's a skill or a language you've wanted to learn for a while, an instrument you started to learn to play and gave up on years ago; maybe you already enjoy taking pictures and want to learn more by studying photography and enroll in an online course at a community college. Through a variety of different activities, you can find ways to better align your interests with your intellectual sense of well-being. As you explore and become stronger and more confident in your intellectual sense of well-being, this can improve other dimensions of wellness, such as opening up social circles — whom you hang around with and different people who can contribute to your intellectual wellness and overall sense of well-being.

Social

If you stop to think about the persons you spend most of your leisure time with, what are the activities you usually do with them? If you find that some of your closest friends only care to meet you at the bar, play video games, ask you for favors, or just like to call you and complain or vent their problems, then maybe some of these relationships are more detrimental to your social well-being than helpful. Furthermore, if your only contact with your friends is via social media, perhaps this is a sign that there is some room for improvement in your social well-being. Maybe you can benefit in other dimensions of wellness if you make it a point to more regularly plan events with friends, meet them for dinner, invite them over for a game night, or even seek other groups of people with interests similar to yours. In most cities there are different organizations (e.g. Meetup) that make it easy to find a variety of different groups of like-minded individuals, regardless of what your unique interests are.

Have you ever volunteered? Maybe you volunteered once or twice in the past and forgot how rewarding this can be. This is a wonderful way to meet people with similar interests, similar values, or simply to meet people that you gain inspiration and ideas from in your pursuit of improving your wellness. Volunteering also helps build character and provides an opportunity to meet all sorts of people you wouldn't likely get the chance to meet otherwise.

Although every family has its own unique challenges or family dynamics, don't forget to recognize the significance of relationships with family members for your social well-being. Whether for the positive or negative, relationships with family factor into your social wellness. Many people hold grudges or resentment towards certain family members because of things that were done in the past. However, it's not good for you or your family members to continue to hold onto such grudges. Depending on the situation, it may not be always easy or even possible in some situations, but understand the importance of discussing any of these fallouts or disagreements with each other. For some, confronting disagreements in a respectful manner with fellow family members may be an important step in improving one's sense of social wellness.

Occupational

Do you find purpose or fulfillment in the work you do? Does your work align with your values, your beliefs, and interests? Do you allow yourself adequate time away from work responsibilities to find a fair "work-life balance"? Unfortunately, too many people would answer "no" to these questions. Frankly, not everybody will find a great sense of purpose or fulfillment in their work and that is okay. However, there are different ways to find more joy in the work you do. Besides your primary source of employment and what you do most days of the week, occupational wellness also includes hobbies, volunteer work, or even promotion opportunities that you look forward to in the future with your current employer.

If you find that your sense of occupational well-being is not as strong as other dimensions of wellness, you can improve this area by being more intentional with your time and participate more in activities that contribute to your sense of purpose. For example, seek out volunteer opportunities with non-profit organizations that support causes that you believe in and that you wish to make a difference on the same issue. There are many organizations and groups of people that would love to work with you and benefit from your service. Volunteering with organizations is also a great way to meet new people (helps social wellness) and network with other people that can help open the door to other opportunities that may enhance your occupational and financial well-being in the future. If you've never volunteered before, that is okay — it's never too late to start and reap the endless benefits you may discover by dedicating your time to the service of others.

If you feel a general lack of purpose or fulfillment at work, maybe this is an indication that it's a perfect time to research what really interests you. Or perhaps re-develop skills you have not practiced in a long time, or discover and actualize what skills you would like to develop. As you think more critically about what interests you, sparks your passion or sense of purpose, this can help to identify other employment opportunities to explore and find pathways to adopt new skills and put into practice that you can make a career out of. On the other hand, for people who work too much, the first step to improving occupational wellness might be to reduce work hours and allow more time for balance in the other dimensions of wellness.

Environmental

It is important to feel a sense of security in your own personal environment and consequently, a lack of feeling safe or not being in an environment that supports one's well-being can have an impact on overall wellness. Environmental wellness reflects the condition of the areas where you work, play, learn, and live. Do you spend most of your time in areas that are pleasant and stimulate other interests and dimensions of wellness? Do you spend enough time outdoors, in nature, and other comforting environments that bring you joy? Do you like to reduce, reuse, and recycle your consumer goods and waste? If so, does your environment make this choice convenient and support your value of practicing this responsibility? Do you have easy access to public transportation? Does your environment provide adequate space and safety to encourage learning, relaxation, and contemplation? These are important questions to consider when reflecting on your environmental wellness.

The sense of security and environmental wellness not only includes feeling free from physical harm but also includes easy access to healthy foods, clean air, and water. Many Americans are "food insecure" and do not have convenient access to fresh and healthy food. This is sometimes referred to as living in a "food desert." Estimates suggest approximately 4% of people in the U.S. who live in low-income areas live at least one mile away from the nearest supermarket, and many of these people don't have a car or transportation to get to the supermarket. There are plenty of studies that find a strong link between limited access to fresh, healthy staple foods — fruits, vegetables, whole grains, and lean proteins —and low intake of nutritious foods.[16] Furthermore, as you have learned in this book, this lack of eating nutritious foods is likely to contribute to health problems when the only convenient options for foods are fast foods and other highly processed foods (chips, candy, cupcakes, sodas, and processed meats) from convenience stores.

Financial

Although it's often claimed that money can't buy happiness, not having enough income or access to financial resources when in need can undoubtedly increase stress and sometimes even have a harmful effect on your physical and mental health. Do you usually earn enough to pay your bills on time? If so, do you earn enough to afford non-essential things that bring you joy and value? This dimension of wellness not only reflects overall satisfaction with income, debt, and savings, but it also reflects your understanding of financial measures and access to resources (in other words, financial literacy). If you answered "no" to one or both of these questions, maybe your financial wellness can use some work.

Are student debt or too many maxed-out credit cards some of your main financial concerns? Or, maybe you "make good money, but spend even better money" and always find it difficult to pay bills on time and stress out about this a lot. Do you have a budget established? If so, are you following it? These are important questions to consider when reflecting on your financial wellness. If you don't already have a plentiful amount of savings to cover current living expenses and retirement, or you've grown up without much financial literacy, or you simply don't know how much money is coming in (income) and how much money is going out (expenses) each month, there is a good chance that you will experience financial stress (if not already under such stress).

If limited or lack of income is the primary concern, update your resume and seek out relevant volunteer opportunities to improve or develop networking skills. Consider seeking other employment prospects or find a new skill that can open future employment opportunities.

Spiritual

This dimension of wellness includes a broad interpretation of different ways people can exercise their spirituality. Generally speaking, spirituality is unique to the individual and can reflect personal beliefs and values. This sense of spirituality helps to provide a sense of purpose, meaning, and peace. Although religion is sometimes regarded as interchangeable with spirituality, attending religious services and following religious teachings or practices are not the only ways to exercise this dimension. Spiritual wellness might involve exploring other religions and belief systems with the hope of increasing respect, empathy, and understanding for their companions or fellow community members. Apart from religion, spirituality may be determined from life experiences rather than reflective of religious doctrine studied and what was practiced earlier in life.

Beyond these more obvious ways of exercising spirituality, consider the power of music. The works of renowned author and neurologist, Oliver Sacks help us appreciate the amazing ability of music to elicit a wide array of emotions and memories.[17] Dr. Sacks observed that more area of the brain is stimulated from listening to music than is used to process and understand language. Although many people might not think of music as being spiritual, given how much of our brain is used to process music, it's not too far of a stretch to imagine how music can be a pathway to spirituality.

Given that writing a book can sometimes feel like a daunting and tiring process, there are a couple of musical artists, in particular, that helped to keep me focused and motivated for hours on end. At the start of writing this book, I was just learning to love jazz music. Quite the contrast from the heavy metal and punk rock music (mostly, not exclusively) that I grew up loving — and still enjoy. Looking back, I estimate that well over half the hours that I spent writing, I was listening to, and falling in love with, the whole body of music played by John Coltrane and Miles Davis. These two are musical and artistic geniuses. Their expression and evolution as musicians and as artists seemed to keep me inspired to explore a creative side of my mind and to write more effectively. One might even argue that these artists evolved in their careers to intentionally express themselves more spiritually through music. Even generations later, this music influences listeners like myself and may even have a spiritual impact.

Whether or not you grew up in a religious home or with spiritually-oriented people, you need to take the time to identify what your values and your religious or spiritual beliefs mean to you. Are you tolerant and respectful of other people's beliefs that don't align with yours? If you find it difficult to answer these questions, maybe this is an indication that you can do some work to improve this dimension of wellness. One way to work on reflecting and improving your spiritual well-being is to seek out community resources and groups that enable you to practice spiritual beliefs. For some, this might be finding a new church or seeking a non-denominational place of worship that is more accepting of different beliefs. For others, this might mean finding a safe and peaceful place such as a park or library to practice meditation and personal reflection or even just a calm and peaceful place.

RESOURCES

GENERAL MENTAL HEALTH SERVICES
ADAA Online Support Group – Anxiety and Depression Association of America – https://adaa.org/adaa-online-support-group

Crisis Text Line – Text NAMI to 741-741

NAMI Helpline – National Alliance on Mental Health – 1-800-950-NAMI (6264), NAMI.org

National Institute of Mental Health – www.nimh.nih.gov

National Suicide Prevention Lifeline – 1-800-273-TALK (8255), suicidepreventionlifeline.org

TalkSpace.com – Online and mobile therapy for those looking to connect with a mental health counselor or therapist online

For uninsured or under-insured – National Association of Free & Charitable Clinics – Nafcclinics.org/find-clinic

HELPFUL RESOURCES

DASH Diet Planning Tool – also find DASH eating plans for various caloric needs
https://www.nhlbi.nih.gov/health-topics/dash-eating-plan

IBS Diet and Symptoms Diary- https://www.hopkinsmedicine.org/gastroenterology_hepatology/_pdfs/small_large_intestine/ibd-printable-diet-symptom-diary.pdf

Mental Health America – fast, simple screening tests for different mental health disorders
Https://screening.mhanational.org

Office of Dietary Supplements from the National Institutes of Health –find detailed fact sheets on vitamins, minerals, and other dietary supplements - https://ods.od.nih.gov

Oldways Cultural Food Traditions: A Food and Nutrition Nonprofit Helping People Live Healthier, Happier Lives – learn more about Mediterranean Diet and other traditional diets you might want to model your diet on - https://oldwayspt.org

Sleep diary– found at sleepeducation.org –
http://sleepeducation.org/docs/default-document-library/sleep-diary.pdf

The Anti-Inflammatory Lifestyle Patient Handout by UW Integrative Health – includes a "quick guide to the anti-inflammatory lifestyle" for easy reference - https://www.fammed.wisc.edu/files/webfm-uploads/documents/outreach/im/handout_ai_diet_patient.pdf

RECOMMENDED PHONE APPS

Dr. Greger's Daily Dozen – simple way to track a dozen different foods to eat or behaviors to practice daily "for optimal health and longevity"

Monash University FODMAP Diet – Researchers at Monash University developed this diet. This app does have a cost but provides a guide for following this diet and includes over 70 low FODMAP recipes

My Symptoms Food Diary & Symptom Tracker – simplifies process and provides structure for food elimination trials along with gastrointestinal symptom tracking.

RECOMMENDED PODCASTS

Funk'tional Nutrition Podcast with Erin Holt – integrative and functional nutritionist covering a wide variety of different topics on overall health and functional nutrition

Nutrition Facts Podcast with Michael Greger, M.D., FACLM – found at NutritionFacts.org; author of best-selling nutrition book *How Not to Die*

Nutrition Rewired – by registered dietitian, Erin Kenney, who specializes in digestive health, sports nutrition, mental health, and medical cannabis use

Tiny Leaps, Big Changes with Gregg Clunis – ideas, tips and strategies to help find "progress, not perfect"

Your Nutrition Prescription – by Adrian Chavez, a PhD in physical activity, nutrition and wellness, who breaks down scientific details and teaches you about holistic nutrition and gut-health

RECOMMENDED READING
Additional books about gut-health, nutrition for mental health, or other related-material

Barnard, Dr. Neal D. *Power Foods for the Brain: An Effective 3-Step Plan to Protect Your Mind and Strengthen Your Memory.* New York, NY: Grand Central Publishing, 2013.

Campbell, T. Colin, and Thomas M. Campbell II. *The China Study: The Most Comprehensive Study of Nutrition Ever Conducted and the Startling Implications for Diet, Weight Loss and Long-Term Health.* Jackson, TN: BenBella Books, 2006.

Greger, Michael. *How Not to Die: Discover the Foods Scientifically Proven to Prevent and Reverse Disease.* New York, NY: Flatiron Books, 2015.

Junger, Dr. Alejandro. *Clean Gut: The Breakthrough Plan for Eliminating the Root Cause of Disease and Revolutionizing Your Health.* New York, NY: HarperCollins Publishers, 2013.

Korn, Leslie E. *Nutrition Essentials for Mental Health: A Complete Guide to the Food-Mood Connection.* New York, NY: W.W. Norton & Company, 2016.

Mancinelli, K. *The Ketogenic Diet - The Scientifically Proven Approach to Fast, Healthy Weight Loss.* Berkeley, CA: Ulysses Press, 2015.

Menzel P, D'Aluisio F. *Hungry Planet: What the World Eats.* Napa CA: Material World Books, 2007.

Miller, Ali. *The Anti-Anxiety Diet: A Whole-Body Program to Stop Racing Thoughts, Banish Worry and Live Panic-Free.* Berkeley, CA: Ulysses Press, 2018.

Mullin, Gerard E. *The Gut Balance Revolution: Boost Your Metabolism, Restore Your Inner Ecology, and Lose the Weight for Good.* New York, NY: Rodale Inc., 2015.

Naidoo, Uma. *This is Your Brain on Food: An Indispensable Guide to the Surprising Foods that Fight Depression, Anxiety, PTSD, OCD, ADHD and More.* New York, NY: Little, Brown Spark, 2020

Willett, Walter, *Eat, Drink, and Be Healthy: The Harvard School to Healthy Eating.* New York: Simon & Schuster, 2001.

COOKBOOKS FOR HEALTHFUL EATING

Family Friendly Mediterranean-style Cooking with a Groundbreaking Guide to Weight Loss, Weight Control and Cardiovascular Health by Arnold Slyper. Targum Publishers, Jerusalem, 2017.

Healthy Heart, Healthy Planet: Delicious Plant-Based Recipes and Tips to Reduce Heart Disease, Lose Weight, and Preserve the Environment by Dr. Cathi Misquitta and Dr. Rajiv Misquitta. CreateSpace; South Carolina, 2014.

Rewire Your Gut: Recipes to Heal Your Gut and Improve Your Health by Erin Kenney, MS, RDN, HCP, 2019.

Rewire Your Sweet Tooth: Delectable Creations to Support a Healthy Gut by Erin Kenney, MS, RDN, HCP, 2020.

The Complete Anti-Inflammatory Diet for Beginners: A No-Stress Meal Plan with Easy Recipes to Heal the Immune System by Dorothy Calimeris and Lulu Cook. Rockridge Press, Berkeley, CA, 2017.

The Easy 5 Ingredient Pescatarian Cookbook: Simple Recipes for Delicious, Heart-Healthy Meals by Andy DeSantis and Michelle Anderson. Rockridge Press, Emeryville, CA, 2019.

WEBSITES
Miscellaneous resources, support, and information to help with lifestyle changes
AboutIBS.org – find information, support, and other resources at this site managed by the International Foundation for Gastrointestinal Disorders

BlueZones.com – from meal planning to recipes, or visit to learn more about the Blue Zones Power 9, the common lifestyle habits shared among these widely-known healthy populations

ChangeDirection.org – campaign to help fight the stigma of mental health and advancing, changing the conversation about mental health

Clubhouse-Intl.org – Clubhouse International is a network of support that fosters community and "helps start and grow Clubhouses globally, where people with mental illness can go to get their lives back."

DiaTribe.org – DiaTribe Foundation is a source of support, advocacy and other resources for those with — or caregivers of those with — diabetes or prediabetes.

EWG.org – Environmental Working Group provides information and research to help inform consumers to live in a healthier environment. This organization established the "Dirty Dozen" and the "Clean Fifteen" lists of the twelve produce items most heavily sprayed with pesticides and fifteen produce items least sprayed with pesticides

ForksOverKnives.com – from books, films, magazines, to recipes and meal planner tools, success stories, and cooking courses, ForksOverKnives.com provides a wealth of resources for those looking to transition to a whole-foods plant-based diet

Gastro.org – American Gastroenterological Association is an international non-profit organization, a society of gastrointestinal (GI) health experts who are dedicated to advancing the science and understanding of complex GI disorders.

JEDfoundation.org – The JED Foundation is a non-profit organization for teens and young adults that helps protect emotional health and emphasizes suicide prevention.

Ketonutrition.org – all things keto, from books, blogs, and podcasts, you can also find a lot of research and learn more about the science behind the ketogenic diet

LocalHarvest.org – online directory of local farms, farmers markets, and other community produce resources such as community supported agriculture (CSAs) and pick-your-own produce businesses

MeatlessMonday.com – educational campaign to help people gradually transition to vegetarian or whole-foods plant-based diet

Meetup.com – website/service used for connecting to and meeting up with like-minded individuals, with any similar topics of interest. If there isn't already a group existing that you're looking for, create one and be the group leader!

NutritionFacts.org – learn about different nutrition topics, hear what the latest science says about current hot topics in nutrition. In other words, this site is "a strictly non-commercial, science-based public service."

NutritionStudies.org – nonprofit organization "committed to increasing awareness of the extraordinary impact that food has on the health of our bodies, our communities, and our planet"

PCRM.org – Physicians Committee for Responsible Medicine is a hub of resources for those transitioning to a whole-foods plant-based diet, or in their words, "leading a revolution in medicine that puts a new focus on health and compassion."

PlantBasedDocs.com – global directory of educational tools on whole-foods plant-based diet and directory of plant-based healthcare providers

Plantstrong.com – whole foods, plant-based resources from recipes and blogs, to challenges and events

SeafoodWatch.org (phone app also available) – program created from Monterey Bay Aquarium to inform consumers about making more sustainable and healthful choices when choosing seafood.

SugarScience.UCSF.edu – check out this site if you're looking to learn more about the impact of excess sugar on health

TheGutHealingCommunity.com – resource for those looking for online support, this website has a growing community and collective of all things gut-health

VRG.org (vegetarian research group)- another hub of resources for those looking to eat a vegetarian or vegan diet

Watercheck.com – home water testing kits available for purchase should you care to test your water to see if there is presence, and what the levels are, of toxic metals, viruses, or other volatile organic molecules in your city water or well water

GLOSSARY

ABC

ADD/ADHD attention deficit and attention deficit hyperactivity disorders are chronic conditions, usually beginning in childhood, that include difficulty concentrating, impulsiveness, and hyperactivity

Allergen a substance — usually a protein, if a food allergen — that triggers the immune system to signal an inflammatory reaction

Allergy an immune response to a particular substance in food or the environment that results in inflammation, ranging in severity from annoying to life-threatening

Amino acids biological building blocks of protein and end products of protein digestion; 20 amino acids ("essential amino acids") are necessary for human metabolism and growth and must be supplied by food

Antioxidants substances found in foods that help prevent excess oxidation and protect the body from cellular damage that normally occurs throughout life

Anxiety a vague, uneasy feeling of discomfort or dread

Autoimmune describes the body's loss of tolerance for an internal cellular substance triggering an inflammatory response typically reserved as a defense against attack from external pathogens

Autonomic nervous system part of the nervous system that is not within conscious control, and automatically regulates bodily functions such as breathing, heartrate, and digestion

Biochemistry the chemistry of living things

Bifidobacteria a group of bacteria (probiotics) that benefit the human host, such as promoting normal digestion and limiting risks to infection from other harmful bacteria

B-vitamins a group of vitamins that are water-soluble and serve important roles in metabolism such as releasing energy from carbohydrates and fats

Biofilm a layer of bacteria that adheres to a surface or lining of the intestines, for example, and may require special enzymes to get rid of

Bipolar disorders a mental health disorder marked by alternating between states of mania and depression

Cardiovascular concerning the heart and blood vessels

Chronic obstructive pulmonary disease (COPD) a type of lung disease that disrupts airflow and increases difficulty of breathing

Clinical trial a carefully designed and executed research study that investigates the safety and effectiveness of medications, foods, or other treatments in individuals

Coenzyme an enzyme activator

Complementary and integrative medicine (CIM) used along with conventional medical care and including integrated forms of holistic care

Cortisol a type of stress hormone produced by the adrenal glands and helps regulate which type of macronutrient —carbohydrates, fats, or proteins — are used to meet energy demands

Cross-sectional study a review of data describing a specific segment of the population at a specific time or period of time

Cytokines type of protein produced primarily by white blood cells and related to the immune system

DEF

Depression a chronic condition marked by poor mood, sadness, hopelessness, and often accompanied by difficulty (or excessive) sleeping and trouble with concentrating

Diverticula abnormally formed pouches within the colon. Although diverticula are common, they're only considered harmful once they become inflamed and then are diagnosed as diverticulitis

DNA short for deoxyribonucleic acid, chemical name for biological compound that carries genetic information in all living organisms

Dopamine a neurotransmitter or brain messenger produced in different areas of the brain and synthesized by bacteria in the intestinal tract; used in the nervous system to help regulate emotions

Dysbiosis an imbalance of different types of bacteria in areas, especially the gut, that otherwise would contribute health benefits to the human host, i.e. too much bad bacteria in the gut and not enough "good gut bugs"

Electrolytes essential minerals in the diet that have an electrical charge and are important for normal functioning of the heart, blood pressure, nervous system, and muscle function

Enteric nervous system part of the nervous system that is responsible for governing the function of the gastrointestinal (GI) tract and communication between the brain and GI tract

Enterocytes the main type of cell that comprise the lining of the intestinal tract

Enzyme an organic catalyst; a protein that speeds up the rate of biochemical reactions in a cell

Epidemiology the branch of science that explores relationships between large populations of people and health outcomes, especially long-term health outcomes

Epidemiological study collection of data to determine the distribution and determinants of health in populations for the purpose of managing infectious diseases and health-related environmental conditions

Essential fatty acids (EFAs) a type of nutrient that is required for normal health, but is not produced in the human body, therefore must be provided in the diet for good health

Fasting the practice of abstaining from eating or drinking any calorie-containing beverages for an extended period of time

Fasting-mimicking diet (FMD) a diet that restricts daily caloric intake to less than half a normal day's calories which can have similar effects on the metabolism as fasting

Fiber indigestible parts of foods that serve important roles for digestive and immune health

FODMAP short for fermentable, oligo-, di-, mono-saccharides and polyols; these are different types of carbohydrates and fibers that tend to produce more gas in those with irritable bowel syndrome

Folate one of the B-vitamins (B-9); form of the vitamin found naturally in foods; considered in its "reduced form"

Folic acid the form of vitamin B-9 found in fortified foods and in dietary supplements; considered in its "oxidized form"

Food allergy an atypical response to a food, usually a particular protein, that causes the immune system to react

Food intolerance also referred to as a food sensitivity, refers to a variety of unpleasant symptoms experienced by a person when eating particular foods they are unable to digest properly

Fructose a simple sugar, found naturally in fruits and commercially produced to add to processed food products; unlike glucose that can be processed by all cells, fructose must be processed by the liver

Functional medicine a type of alternative medicine practice that includes a variety of holistic methods and treatments

GHI

GABA gamma-aminobutyric acid, an important neurotransmitter, that helps promote relaxation and a healthy nervous system

Gastritis inflammation of the stomach lining

Gastrointestinal concerning the stomach and the intestinal tract

Gastroparesis medical condition where the normal function and movement of the stomach muscle is disrupted, commonly associated with nausea and vomiting

GERD gastroesophageal reflux disease, a chronic condition marked by acid reflux and heartburn

Glucose a simple sugar found in fruits and other plants; the end product of carbohydrate digestion

Gut common term for stomach and the intestines, both small intestine and large intestine

Gut-barrier includes the physical barrier composed of enterocytes and tight junctions between them, also includes protective gut bacteria and a layer of mucus

H. pylori a type of bacteria commonly found in the stomach of humans; some evidence shows this type of bacteria may have health benefits for some people

High fructose corn syrup (HFCS) a commercially produced sweetener, with a higher proportion of fructose to glucose, this gives a sweeter taste compared to using more glucose

Highly processed food products (HPFPs) food products that are commercially produced with a lot of processed oils, grains, added sugars, and also tend to include a variety of artificial flavors, colors, and/or preservatives; tend to be higher in calories and lower in essential nutrients

Holistic an approach that involves consideration of all interconnected parts and potential diagnoses; can also be referred to as a whole-person model of care

Homeostasis a state of stable, relatively normal or healthy balance or range of physiological processes in the body

Homocysteine an amino acid, a natural byproduct of certain biochemical reactions in the body

Hormone a substance originating in an organ or body part that is conveyed through the blood to another body part, chemically stimulating that part to increase or decrease functional activity or to increase or decrease secretion of another hormone

Hydration concerning water and fluid needs and intake

Hypermetabolic a state where the metabolism is operating at a much faster than normal rate, significantly increasing calorie and protein needs

Hypoglycemia low blood sugars, below what is considered within a normal healthy range

HPA-axis hypothalamic-pituitary-adrenal axis is the body's stress control system; a coordination between certain areas of the brain and adrenal glands that sit on top of the kidneys; this activates the "fight or flight" response

Inflammation a protective reaction of the immune system — may be acute in a localized area, or chronic in a broader area of the body; marked by swelling, redness, and pain

Inflammatory bowel diseases (IBD) a chronic condition where sections of the digestive tract are inflamed; this includes ulcerative colitis and Crohn's disease

Insulin a hormone produced in the pancreas, required to stimulate the absorption of blood sugar by cells

Intestines the small intestine and the large intestine, major components of the gastrointestinal tract

Integrated Functional Medicine (IFM) combines conventional methods of medicine such as medications along with other forms of alternative and holistic care

Intestinal permeability (IP) refers to a condition of the intestinal wall that allows food- and other non-food particles to pass into the bloodstream when they are not supposed to

Irritable bowel syndrome (IBS) a chronic gastrointestinal condition marked by gas, constipation, diarrhea, and abdominal pain

JKL

Ketogenic concerning a metabolic state where the body is burning fat as a primary source of energy, rather than carbohydrates, the body's usual and preferred source of energy

Ketone produced in the body from dietary fats as a backup source of fuel when dietary intake of carbohydrates is inadequate

Ketosis metabolic state where the body is producing higher amounts of ketones

Lactose specific type of sugar found naturally in milk and other dairy products; may not be well-tolerated by some people (lactose intolerance)

Lipids refers to different fatty acids, various fats and oils, from foods in the diet

MNO

Macronutrients carbohydrates, proteins and dietary fats; source of all calories from foods

Magnesium mineral element found mostly in our bones and derived from foods such as whole grains, fruits and vegetables

Melatonin a hormone that influences sleep-wake cycles and other circadian rhythms

Meta-analysis type of research study that combines the data from a number of different studies on the same topic to find a consensus or different trends in existing studies

Metabolic acidosis condition in which excessive acid accumulates in the body fluids

Metabolism total of chemical reactions that occur within the body to maintain life

Metabolomics branch of science that studies the cellular and chemical end-products of metabolism

Metformin medication commonly used to control blood sugar levels and treat diabetes

Microbes microscopic organisms, also referred to as microorganisms; includes bacteria, fungi, viruses, and protozoa

Microbiome the community of different microbes living in a particular area of the body; e.g., gut microbiome

Micronutrients nutrients that are required in very small amounts for normal health and growth

Mindfulness state of consciously being aware of something in the moment

Monounsaturated fats certain type of essential fatty acid found in foods, characterized by one double bond in the chain of carbon atoms; required for health

Motility the ability to automatically move; refers to the sequential contractions and movements of the gastrointestinal tract required for normal digestion and absorption

Neurogenesis refers to the ability of nerve cells to develop and regrow

Neurons nerve cells that connect to one another and help to communicate messages between the brain and other areas of the body

Neuropsychiatry scientific discipline that combines the studies on neurological and psychiatric illnesses

Neurotransmitters chemical substance released by neurons that transfers nerve impulses from cell to cell, and helps "communicate" messages between the brain and other parts of the nervous system

NSAIDs non-steroidal anti-inflammatory drugs

Nutrient-dense per calorie, high in vitamins and minerals

Nutrigenomics branch of science that studies the interaction between nutrition, food choices, and the effects on genes and genetic expression

Omega-3 (omega-3 fatty-acids) certain types of polyunsaturated fats that have anti-inflammatory effects

Oxidative stress refers to a state in which excess oxidants are produced in the body and may contribute to cellular damage

PQR

Pathogens microorganisms, or other biological agents, that cause diseases or viruses

Peptic ulcers condition in which the lining of the stomach develops a sore and causes pain

Physiological concerning body function

Phytonutrients substance derived from plants that is believed to have health benefits when consumed

Polyphenols a class of phytonutrients that have protective antioxidant effects

Polyunsaturated fats certain type of essential fatty acids found in certain foods, characterized by two or more double bonds in the chain of carbon atoms; required for health

Potassium mineral element, important for heart health, nerve cell and muscular function, derived from foods such as fruits and vegetables

Probiotics a variety of different strains of bacteria and yeasts that naturally live on and inside humans and have beneficial effects on health

Protein a food component comprised of amino acids; one of the three macronutrients that provides calories and is essential for health

Proton-pump inhibitors ("PPIs") group of medications that reduce symptoms of acid reflux/GERD by decreasing how much stomach acid is produced

Randomized-controlled trial (RCT; study type) an experimental study to assess the effects of a particular drug or treatment in which study participants are assigned randomly to an experimental, a placebo or a control group

Recommended Dietary Allowance (RDA) amounts of different nutrients estimated to be sufficient for the vast majority of healthy people

STUV

Saturated fats type of dietary fat that is considered less healthy

Selenium essential mineral important for health; has antioxidant-like protective effects

Serotonin a chemical or neurotransmitter that helps send signals between nerve cells; important for digestion, sleep, and mood

SIBO small intestinal bacterial overgrowth; occurs when certain strains of harmful bacteria overgrow in areas where they should not

SIFO small intestinal fungal overgrowth; occurs when strains of fungi grow excessively in areas that they shouldn't in such high concentrations

Sleep apnea also referred to as obstructive sleep apnea, a condition where normal breathing pattern is disrupted during sleep resulting in less oxygen delivered to the brain and other cells of the body

Standard American Diet (SAD) daily food consumption consists primarily of "ultra-processed" food products, high in refined grains, added sugars, salt and other unhealthy ingredients and lacking essential nutrients

Supplements products that are ingested with the intent of complementing one's diet and providing more of certain nutrients that may be lacking in the diet

Sympathetic nervous system division of the nervous system important for helping regulate stress levels, heart rate, and blood vessels

Tryptophan an essential amino acid, important for producing hormones and neurotransmitters, such as melatonin and serotonin

WXYZ

Whole foods unprocessed, or minimally processed, foods

Zinc essential mineral important for immune system health and found in foods such as certain types of seafood, red meats, and lesser amounts in dairy, poultry, and pork

Zonulin type of protein that affects the tight junctions between intestinal cells, increased levels can lead to increased intestinal permeability

NOTES

Introduction

[1] Sathyanarayana TS et al. Understanding nutrition, depression and mental illnesses. *Indian J Psychiatry*, 2008, 50(2):77-82.

[2] Greenblatt J.M. and Brogan K. Integrative Therapies for Depression: Redefining Models for Assessment, Treatment, and Prevention. Boca Raton FL: Taylor & Francis Group, 2016.

[3] Mullin GE. *The Gut Balance Revolution: Boost Your Metabolism, Restore Your Inner Ecology, and Lose the Weight For Good.* New York NY: Rodale Inc., 2015.

[4] Food and Nutrition Board of the Institute of Medicine, National Academy of Sciences https://ods.od.nih.gov/HealthInformation/Dietary_Reference_Intakes. aspx.

[5] National Alliance on Mental Illness. https://www.NAMI.org/# Accessed December 2019.

[6] National Institute of Mental Health. https://www.nimh.nih.gov/health/statistics/ mental-illness.shtml Accessed March 2020.

[7] National Alliance on Mental Illness. https://www.NAMI.org/# Accessed December 2019.

[8] Greenblatt and Brogan. opus cit.

[9] American Foundation for Suicide Prevention. Suicide Statistics. https://afsp.org/ about-suicide/suicide-statistics/ Accessed March 2020.

[10] Greenblatt and Brogan. opus cit.

Chapter 1

[1] Grosso G et al. Role of omega-3 fatty acids in the treatment of depressive orders: A comprehensive meta-analysis of randomized clinical trials. *PLOS One.* 2014 9(5):1-18.

[2] Galland L. The Gut Microbiome and the Brain. *J Med Food.* 2014, 17(12):1261-1272.

[3] Miller Ali. *The Anti Anxiety Diet: A Whole Body Program to Stop Racing Thoughts, Banish Worry and Live Panic-Free.* Berkeley CA: Ulysses Press, 2018.

[4] American Psychiatric Association *Diagnostic and Statistical Manual of Mental Disorders-IV.*

[5] Lakhan SE and Vieira, KF. Nutritional therapies for mental disorders. *Nutrition Journal.* 2008, 7:2 (Review)

[6] Dipasquale S et al. The dietary pattern of patients with schizophrenia: A systematic review. *J Psychiatr Res.* 2013, 47 (2):197-207.

[7] Brish R et al. The role of dopamine in schizophrenia from a neurobiological and evolutionary perspective: old fashioned, but still in vogue. *Front Psychiatry.* 2014, 5(47):1-11.

[8] Preston J and Johnson J. Clinical Psychopharmacology Made Ridiculously Simple. (8th edition update for DSM-V). Miami FL: MedMaster Inc., 2019.

[9] Aucoin M and LaChance L. Vitamin B12, vitamin B6, folic acid and psychosis: A review. *J Orthomol Med.* 2018, 33 (5).

[10] Firth J et al. Nutritional deficiencies and clinical correlates in first-episode psychosis: A systematic review and meta-analysis. *Schizophren Bull.* 2017, 44(6):1275-1292.

[11] Korn L. Nutrition Essentials for Mental Health: A Complete Guide to the Food-Mood Connection. New York NY: W.W. Norton & Company Inc., 2016.

[12] Lakhan and Viera, opus cit.

[13] Grosso, G, et .al. opus cit.

[14] Bloch MH and Hannestad J. Omega-3 fatty acids for the treatment of depression: Systematic review and meta-analysis. *Mol Psychiatry.* 2012, 17(12):1272-1282.

[15] Eby GA and Eby KL. Rapid recovery from major depression using magnesium treatment. *Medical Hypotheses.* 2006, 67(2):362-370.

[16] National Institutes of Health Office of Dietary Supplements. Fact Sheet for Health Professionals. https://ods.od.nih.gov/factsheets/Calcium-HealthProfessional/ Accessed February 2020.

[17] Stanislawska M et al. The severity of depressive symptoms vs. serum Mg and Zn Levels in postmenopausal women. *Biol Trace Elem Res.* 2014, 157:30-35.

[18] Gu Y et al. Association between serum magnesium levels and depression in stroke patients. *Aging Dis.* 2016, 7:687-690.

[19] Jacka FN et al. Association between magnesium intake and depression and anxiety in community-dwelling adults: the Hordaland Health Study. *Aust N Z J Psychiatry.* 2009, 43(1):45-52.

[20] Tarleton EK and Littenberg B. Magnesium intake and depression in adults. *J Am Board Fam Med.* 2015, 28:249–256.

[21] National Institutes of Health, Office of Dietary Supplements. Fact Sheet for Health Professionals. https://ods.od.nih.gov/factsheets/Zinc-HealthProfessional/ Accessed February 2020.

[22] Wang J et al. Zinc, magnesium, selenium and depression: A review of the evidence, potential mechanisms and implications. *Nutrients.* 2018, 10 (584):1-19.

Chapter 2

[1] Hunter P. The inflammation theory of disease." European Molecular Biology Organization. 2012, 13(11):968-970.

[2] Causes of Death Collaborators (GBD). Global, regional, and national age-sex-specific mortality for 282 causes of death in 195 countries and territories, 1980–2017: A systematic analysis for the Global Burden of Disease Study 2017. *Lancet* 392, 1736–1788 (2018).

[3] Yang C et al. Inflammatory markers and treatment outcomes in treatment resistant depression: A systematic review. *J Affect Disord.* 2019, 257:640-649.

[4] Greenblatt JM and Brogan K. Integrative Therapies for Depression: Redefining Models for Assessment, Treatment, and Prevention. Boca Raton FL: Taylor & Francis Group, 2016.

[5] Pahwa R et al. Chronic Inflammation. StatPearls Internet. 2019.

[6] Barbosa P. Biomarkers of Aging and Chronic Inflammation. Presented at the 2015 New York Clinical Conference, New York College of Podiatric Medicine.

[7] Galecki P and Talarowska M. Inflammatory theory of depression. *Psychiatria Polska.* 2018, 52(3):437-447.

[8] Raison C and Miller AH. Is depression an inflammatory disorder? *Current Psychiatry Reports.* 2011, 13(6):467-475.

[9] Greenblatt and Brogan, opus cit.

[10] Hall KD, et al. Ultra-processed diets cause excess calorie intake and weight gain: A one-month inpatient randomized controlled trial of ad libitum food intake. *Cell Metabolism.* May 16, 2019.

[11] Lordan R et al. Dairy fats and cardiovascular disease: do we really need to be concerned? *Foods.* 2018, 7(29):1-34.

[12] Siri-Tarino PW et al. Meta-analysis of prospective cohort studies evaluating the association of saturated fat with cardiovascular disease. *Am J Clin Nutr.* 2010, 91:535-546.

Chapter 3

[1] Gershon MD. The enteric nervous system: A second brain. *Hospital Practice.* 1999, 34(7):31-52.

[2] Hadhazy A. Think twice: How the gut's 'second brain' influences mood and well-being. *Scientific American.* https://www.scientificamerican.com/article/gut-second-brain/ Accessed March 2020.

[3] Johns Hopkins Medicine. The brain-gut connection. https://www.hopkinsmedicine.org/health/wellness-and-prevention/the-brain-gut-connection Accessed February 2020.

[4] Korn L. Nutrition Essentials for Mental Health: A Complete Guide to the Food-Mood Connection. W.W. Norton & Company, Inc.: New York NY, 2016.

[5] Blaser MJ. Missing Microbes: How the Overuse of Antibiotics Is Fueling Our Modern Plagues. New York NY: Henry Holt and Company, 2014.

[6] Huang TT et al. Current understanding of gut microbiota in mood disorders: An update of human studies. *Front Genet.* 2019, 10(98):1-12.

[7] Blaser MJ. opus cit.

[8] Vighi, G et al. Allergy and the gastrointestinal system. *J Clin Exp Immunol.* 2008, 153(1): 3-6.b.

[9] Greenblatt JM and Brogan K. Integrative Therapies for Depression: Redefining Models for Assessment, Treatment, and Prevention. Boca Raton FL: Taylor & Francis Group, 2016.

[10] Canny GO and McCormick BA. Bacteria in the intestine, helpful residents or enemies from within? *Infection and Immunity.* 2008, 76(8):3360-3373.

[11] Peng L et al. Effects of butyrate on intestinal barrier function in a Caco-2 cell monolayer model of intestinal barrier. *Pediatr Res.* 2006, 61(1): 37-41.

[12] Cheng LH et al. Psychobiotics in mental health, Neurodegenerative and neurodevelopmental disorders. *Journal of Food and Drug Analysis.* 2019, 27(3):632-848.

[13] Mangiola F et al. Gut microbiota in autism and mood disorders. *World J Gastroenterol.* 2016, 22(1):361-368.

[14] Fasano A. Zonulin and its regulation of intestinal barrier function: The biological door to inflammation, autoimmunity, and cancer. *Physiol Rev.* 2011, 91:151-175.

[15] Fisher S. An Anti-Inflammatory Lifestyle. Institute for Brain Potential, seminar packet. Attended seminar: February 27, 2020.

[16] Peng L et al. opus cit.

[17] Yoshii K et al. Metabolism of dietary and microbial vitamin B family in the regulation of host immunity. *Front Nutr.* 2019, 6(48):1-12.

[18] Galland L The gut microbiome and the brain. *J Med Food.* 2014, 17(12):1261-1272.

[19] Yano JM et al. Indigenous bacteria from the gut microbiota regulate host serotonin biosynthesis. *Cell.* 2015, 161(2):264-276.

[20] Dhakal R, Bajpai VK and Baek KH. Production of GABA by microorganisms: A review. *Brazilian Journal of Microbiology.* 2011, 1230-1241.

[21] Galland L. The gut microbiome and the brain. *J Med Food.* 2014, 17(12):1261-1272.

Chapter 4

[1] Korn L. Nutrition Essentials for Mental Health: A Complete Guide to the Food-Mood Connection. New York NY: W.W. Norton & Company Inc., 2016.

[2] Fasano A. Zonulin and its regulation of intestinal barrier function: The biological door to inflammation autoimmunity, and cancer. *Physiol Rev.* 2011, 91:151-175.

[3] Hollon J. et al. Effect of gliadin on permeability of intestinal biopsy explants from celiac disease patients and patients with non-celiac gluten sensitivity. *Nutrients.* 2015, 7: 1575-1576.

[4] Khalili H. Risk of inflammatory bowel disease with oral contraceptives and menopausal hormone therapy: Current evidence and future directions. *Drug Saf.* 2016;39(3):193-197. doi:10.1007/s40264-015-0372-y

[5] Korn L. opus cit.

[6] Naito Y et al. Intestinal dysbiosis secondary to proton-pump inhibitor use. *Digestion.* 2018, 97:195-204.

[7] Wu H et al. Metformin alters the gut microbiome in individuals with treatment-naive Type-2 diabetes, contributing to the therapeutic effects of the drug. *Nature Medicine.* 2017, 23:850-858.

[8] Johns Hopkins Medicine. Irritable Bowel Syndrome: Introduction https://www.hopkinsmedicine.org/gastroenterology_hepatology/_pdfs/small_large_intestine/irritable_bowel_byndrome_ibs.pdf Accessed April 2020.

[9] Lasalandra M. The Sensitive Gut: What You Can Do to Prevent & Treat Dyspepsia, Reflux Disease, Irritable Bowel Syndrome, Constipation, and More. New York NY: Fireside, 2001.

[10] Sipponen P and Maaroos HI. Chronic gastritis. *Scand J Gastroenterol.* 2015, 50:657-667.

[11] Blaser MJ Missing Microbes: How the Overuse of Antibiotics Is Fueling Our Modern Plagues. New York NY: Henry Holt and Company LLC, 2014.

[12] Lasalandra M. opus cit.

[13] Blaser, opus cit.

[14] Farrell B et al. Deprescribing proton pump inhibitors: evidence-based clinical practice guideline. *Canadian Family Physician.* 2017, 63:354-364.

[15] Mullin GE. The Gut Balance Revolution: Boost Your Metabolism, Restore Your Inner Ecology, and Lose the Weight for Good. New York NY: Rodale Inc., 2015.

[16] Jacobs C et al. Dysmotility and PPI use are independent risk factors for small intestinal bacterial and/or fungal growth. *Aliment Pharmacol Ther.* 2013, 37(11):1103-1111.

[17] Korn L. opus cit.

[18] Mayo Clinic. Food Allergy: Overview. https://www.mayoclinic.org/diseases-conditions/food-allergy/symptoms-causes/syc-20355095 Accessed April 2020.

[19] University of Nebraska-Lincoln. Food Allergy Research and Resource Program. The Big-8. Allergenic Foods and Their Allergens. https://farrp.unl.edu/informallbig8 Accessed April 2020.

[20] Fedewa A and Rao SSC. Dietary fructose intolerance, fructan intolerance and FODMAPs. *Curr Gastrolenterol Rep.* 2014, 16(1):1-13.

[21] Johns Hopkins Medicine. Breath Test. https://www.hopkinsmedicine.org/gastroenterology_hepatology/_forms/patient_info/Breath_test_instructions_updated_6_5_18.pdf Accessed April 2020.

[22] Vighi G et al. Allergy and the gastrointestinal system. *J Clin Exp Immunol.* 2008, 153(1):3-6.

[23] Johns Hopkins Medicine. What are common symptoms of autoimmune disease? https://www.hopkinsmedicine.org/health/wellness-and-prevention/what-are-common-symptoms-of-autoimmune-disease Accessed April 2020.

[24] Fasano A. opus cit.

[25] Duerkop BA et al. Immune responses to the microbiota at the intestinal mucosal surface. *Immunity.* 2009, 31:368-376.

[26] King K. "What is the Low FODMAP diet?" Eat right. Academy of Nutrition and Dietetics. August 2020.

[27]. Hatanaka M. My Global Table: Japan. *Food & Nutrition Magazine.* July/August 2019.

[28] Mullin GE. opus cit.

[29] Leech B et al. Treatment interventions for the management of intestinal permeability: A cross-sectional survey of complementary and integrative medicine practitioners. *J Altern Complement Med.* 2019, 25(6):623-636.

Chapter 5

[1] Patterson RE and Sears DD. Metabolic effects of intermittent fasting. *Annual Review of Nutrition.* 2017, 37:371-93.

[2] Longo VD and Mattson MP. Fasting: Molecular mechanisms and clinical applications. *Cell Metabolism.* 2014, 19(2):181-192.

[3] Antoni R, Johnston KL, Collins AL and Robertson, MD. Effects of intermittent fasting on glucose and lipid metabolism. *Proceedings of the Nutrition Society.* 2017, 76:361-368.

[4] Wolfram T. Investigating intermittent fasting. *Food & Nutrition Magazine.* 2018, September/October: 14-15.

[5] Mattson MP, Longo VD and Harvie M. Impact of intermittent fasting on health and disease processes. *Ageing Res Rev.* 2017, 39:46-58.

[6] Bendix A. Eight signs your intermittent fasting diet has become unsafe or unhealthy. Business Insider. 2019 https://www.businessinsider.com/signs-intermittent-fasting-unsafe-unhealthy-2019-7#it-could-also-makeyou-less-aware-or-alert-3 Accessed February 2020.

[7] London J. What you should know about the 16:8 diet before you start fasting Good Housekeeping Institute, July 14, 2020.

[8] Mosley, Michael. The 5.2 Diet. https://thebloodsugardiet.com/the-52-bsd

[9] Pilon, Brad. https://bradpilon.com/weight-loss/my-philosophy-of-intermittent-fasting/

[10] Trepanowski JF et al. Effect of alternate-day fasting on weight loss, weight maintenance and cardioprotection among metabolically healthy obese adults. *JAMA Internal Medicine.* 2017, 177(7):930-938.

[11] Wei M et al. Fasting-mimicking diet and markers/risk factors for aging, diabetes, cancer, and cardiovascular disease. *Science Translational Medicine.* 2017, 9(377): 1-25.

[12] Sampaio LP. Ketogenic diet for epilepsy treatment. *Arquivos de Neuro-Psiquiatria.* 2016, 74(10):842-848.

[13] Mancinelli K. The Ketogenic Diet: The Scientifically Proven Approach to Fast, Healthy Weight Loss. Berkeley CA: Ulysses Press, 2015.

[14] Gibson AA et al. Do ketogenic diets really suppress appetite? A systematic review and meta-analysis. *Obesity Reviews.* 2015, 16(1):64-76.

[15] Campos M. What is Keto Flu? Boston MA: Harvard Health Publishing, 2018 https://www.health.harvard.edu/blog/what-is-keto-flu-2018101815052 Accessed February 2020.

[16] Sampaio LP. opus cit.

[17] Mancinelli K. opus cit.

[18] U.S. Food and Drug Administration, Dietary Supplement Health and Education Act of 1994, P.L. 103-417

[19] Jiang T. Re-thinking the dietary supplement laws and regulations 14 years after the dietary supplement health and education act implementation. *Int J Food Sci Nutr.* 2009 Jun;60(4):293-301 Epub 2008 Dec 9.PMID: 19085198.

[20] Firth J et al. The efficacy and safety of nutrient supplements in the treatment of mental disorders: A meta-review of meta-analyses of randomized controlled trials. *World Psychiatry.* 2019, 18:308-324.

[21] Mocking RTJ et al. Meta-analysis and meta-regression of omega-3 polyunsaturated fatty acid supplementation for major depressive disorder. *Transl Psychiatry.* 2016, 6(e756):1-6.

[22] Roberts E, Carter, B, Young AH. Caveat emptor: folate in unipolar depressive illness, a systematic review and meta-analysis. *J Psychopharmacol.* 2018, 33:377-384.

[23] National Institutes of Health, Office of Dietary Supplements. Folate Fact Sheet for Consumers. https://ods.od.nih.gov/factsheets/Folate-Consumer/ Accessed March 2020.

[24] Selhub J et al. B vitamins, homocysteine, and neurocognitive function in the elderly. *Am J Clin Nutr.* 2000, 71(suppl):614-620.

[25] Moretti R and Caruso P. The controversial role of homocysteine in neurology: From labs to clinical practice. *Int J Mol Sci.* 2019, 20(231):1-22.

[26] Boyle N.B, Lawton C and Dye L. The effects of magnesium supplementation on subjective anxiety and stress: A systematic review. *Nutrients.* 2017, 9(429):1-22.

[27] Eby G.A and Eby KL. Magnesium for treatment-resistant depression: A review and hypothesis. *Med Hypotheses.* 2010, 74(4):649-660.

[28] Phelan D et al. Magnesium and mood disorders: Systematic review and meta-analysis. *B J Psych Open.* 2018, 4:167-179.

[29] Basharat S et al. Beneficial effects of zinc on reducing severity of depression. *J Psychol Clin Psychiatry.* 2019, 10(4):135-139.

[30] Wang J et al. Zinc, Magnesium, selenium and depression: A review of the evidence, potential mechanisms and implications. *Nutrients.* 2018, 10(584):1-19.

[31] Soh NL and Walter G. Tryptophan and depression: Can diet alone be the answer? *Acta Neuropsychiatrica.* 2018, 13(12):3-11.

[32] Lakhan SE and Vieira KF. Nutritional therapies for mental disorders. *Nutrition Journal.* 2008, 7: 2 (Review).

[33] National Institutes of Health, Office of Dietary Supplements. Probiotics Fact Sheet for Health Professionals. https://ods.od.nih.gov/factsheets/Probiotics-HealthProfessional/ Accessed March 2020.

[34] McFarland LV et al. Strain-Specificity and Disease-Specificity of probiotic efficacy: A systematic review and meta-analysis. *Frontiers in Medicine.* 2018, 5(124).

[35] Sniffen JC et al. Choosing an appropriate probiotic product for your patient: An evidence-based practical guide. *PloS One.* 2018, 13(12): 1-22.

[36] Pirbaglou M et al. Probiotic supplementation can positively affect anxiety and depression symptoms: a systematic review of randomized controlled trials. *Nutr Res.* 2018, 13(12):889-898.

[37] Dashti HM et al. Long-term effects of a ketogenic diet in obese patients. *Exp Clin Cardiol.* 2004, 9(3):200-205.

Chapter 6

[1] Junger A. Clean Gut: The Breakthrough Plan for Eliminating the Root Cause of Disease and Revolutionizing Your Health. New York NY: Harper One, 2013.

[2] Menzel P, D'Aluisio F. Hungry Planet: What the World Eats. Napa CA: Material World Books, 2007.

[3] Buettner D and Skemp S. Blue Zones: Lessons from the world's longest lived. *American Journal of Lifestyle Medicine.* 2016, 10(5):318-321.

[4] Buettner D. Blue Zones. Power 9 – Reverse engineering longevity. https://www. bluezones.com/2016/11/power-9/ Accessed July 2020.

[5] Campbell TC and Campbell TM. The China Study: Startling Implications for Diet, Weight Loss and Long-Term Health. Dallas TX: Benbella Books Inc., 2006.

[6] Ludwig DS, Ebbeling CB, Heymsfield SB. Improving the quality of dietary research. *JAMA.* 2019;322(16):1549–1550. doi:10.1001/jama.2019.11169.

[7] Santesso N et al. Effects of higher versus lower-protein diets on health outcomes: A systematic review and meta-analysis. *European Journal of Clinical Nutrition.* 2012, 66:780-788.

[8] Levine ME et al. Low Protein intake is associated with a major reduction in IGF-1, Cancer, and overall mortality in the 65 and younger but not older population. *Cell Metabolism.* 2014, 19 (3):407-417.

[9] Harvard T. H. Chan School of Public Health Department of Nutrition and The Culinary Institute of America, Menus of Change 2018 Annual Report. https:// www.menusofchange.org/images/uploads/pages/2018_Menus_of_Change_Annual_Report_FINAL.pdf

[10] Pollan M. In Defense of Food. New York NY: Penguin Books, 2008.

Chapter 7

[1] Doran, G. T. (1981). There's a S.M.A.R.T. way to write management's goals and objectives. *Management Review.* 70 (11): 35–36. See https://www.projectsmart. co.uk/brief-history-of-smart-goals.php.

[2] Sacks, Frank M., et al. Effects on blood pressure of reduced dietary sodium and the Dietary Approaches to Stop Hypertension (DASH) diet. *NEJM* 344.1 (2001): 3-10.

[3] U.S. News & World Report. Health: Mediterranean Diet. https://health.usnews. com/best-diet/mediterranean-diet Accessed July 2020.

[4] Harvard Women's Health Watch. Foods That Fight Inflammation. https://www.health.harvard.edu/staying-healthy/foods-that-fight-inflammation.

[5] Academy of Nutrition and Dietetics, EatRight Pro. The MIND Diet. https://www.eatrightpro.org/news-center/nutrition-trends/health-promotion/the-mind-diet Accessed July 2020.

[6] Morris MC et al. MIND Diet associated with reduced incidence of Alzheimer's disease. *Alzheimers Dement.* 2015, 11(9):1007-1014.

[7] _____. MIND Diet slows cognitive decline in aging. *Alzheimers Dement.* 2015, 11(9)1007-1014.

[8] Jacka FN et al. A Randomized controlled trial of dietary improvement for adults with major depression (the SMILES trial). *BMC Medicine.* 2017, 15(23):1-22.

Afterword

[1] Substance Abuse Mental Health Services Administration. Creating a Healthier Life: A Step-By-Step Guide to Wellness. 2016. https://store.samhsa.gov/system/files/sma16-4958.pdf Accessed February 2020.

[2] Harvard Medical School. Sleep and Disease Risk. http://healthysleep.med.harvard.edu/healthy/matters/consequences/sleep-and-disease-risk Accessed March 2020.

[3] National Health, Lung, and Blood Institute. Sleep Science and Sleep Disorders. https://www.nhlbi.nih.gov/science/sleep-science-and-sleep-disorders Accessed March 2019.

[4] Ellis JG et al. The natural history of insomnia: acute insomnia and first-onset depression. *Sleep Journal.* 2014, 37(1):97-106.

[5] American Academy of Sleep Medicine. Sleep Diary. http://sleepeducation.org/docs/default-document-library/sleep-diary.pdf Accessed February 2020.

[6] American Academy of Sleep Medicine. Sleep Habits. http://sleepeducation.org/essentials-in-sleep/healthy-sleep-habits article Accessed February 2020.

[7] Greenblatt JM and Brogan K. Integrative Therapies for Depression: Redefining Models for Assessment, Treatment, and Prevention. Boca Raton FL: Taylor & Francis Group, 2016.

[8] Centers for Disease Control. How Much Sleep Do I Need? https://www.cdc.gov/sleep/about_sleep/how_much_sleep.html Accessed February 2020:

[9] Urponen H et al. Self-evaluations of factors promoting and disturbing sleep: an epidemiological survey in finland. *Social Science & Medicine.* 1988. 26(4): 443-450.

[10] Sharma A et al. Exercise for mental health. Primary Care Companion?? *J Clin Psychiatry.* 2006, 8(2):106.

[11] Holford P. Optimum Nutrition for the Mind, Laguna Beach CA: Basic Health Publications Inc., 2004.

[12] National Institute for Mental Health. Five Things You Should Know About Stress. https://www.nimh.nih.gov/health/publications/stress/index.shtml Accessed February 2020.

[13] Newcomer JW et al. Decreased memory performance in healthy humans induced by stress-level cortisol treatment. *Arch Gen Psychiatry.* 1999, 56(6): 527-533.

[14] Help Guide. Benefits of mindfulness: Practices for improving emotional and physical well-being. (A Harvard Health article) https://www.helpguide.org/harvard/benefits-of-mindfulness.htm Accessed March 2020.

[15] Substance Abuse Mental Health Services Administration, opus cit.

[16] U.S Department of Agriculture, Economic Research Service. Access to Affordable and Nutritious Food: Measuring and Understanding Food Deserts and Their Consequences. (Report Summary).

[17] Sacks, Oliver, Musicophilia: Tales of Music and the Brain. New York NY: Random House, 2007. https://www.oliversacks.com/books-by-oliver-sacks/musicophilia/ Accessed September 2020.

INDEX

Made in the USA
Las Vegas, NV
05 April 2021